T

WHAT IT DOES;
HOW IT CAN GO WRONG;
HOW TO KEEP IT HEALTHY

THE HEART

WHAT IT DOES;
HOW IT CAN GO WRONG;
HOW TO KEEP IT HEALTHY

by

ALASTAIR HUNTER, M.D., F.R.C.P.

PAPERFRONTS
ELLIOT RIGHT WAY BOOKS,
KINGSWOOD, SURREY, U.K.

Made and printed in Great Britain by Love and Malcomson, Redhill, Surrey

CONTENTS

LIST OF ILLUSTRATIONS

To   Dr. A. E. Clark-Kennedy F.R.C.P.
in appreciation.

INTRODUCTION

Doctors are sometimes criticised for not telling patients enough about the nature of their illness, about what has to be done for it and about the likely outcome. In part no doubt this is because it is difficult to express in plain English the technical language in which doctors necessarily think but it is also a consequence of the very limited knowledge which many laymen have of the way in which the body works and how it may go wrong.

This book is not a substitute for doctors and still less is it a do-it-yourself kit for household medicine. It is simply an attempt to make medical advice about your heart more understandable and therefore more useful.

1
WHAT YOUR HEART DOES

SUMMARY

Every part of the body needs blood if it is to work properly. Blood circulates. The heart drives the circulation; it is therefore essential to life. Blood is propelled from the left side of the heart in arteries and carries oxygen and nutrients to the tissues. The tissues use these and form carbon dioxide, water and acid end products in the process. Blood removes these from the tissues before returning in veins to the right side of the heart. From there it is propelled through the lungs, where it is oxygenated and then returned to the left heart for recirculation.

The working of the body depends upon a complex process known as metabolism. Metabolism uses oxygen and breaks down nutrients to supply energy to the body and to maintain the health of the tissues. It is in this process that carbon dioxide, water and other end products, particularly acids, are formed. They have to be removed by the blood and eventually taken to the lungs for reoxygenation, to the liver for reprocessing or to the kidneys for removal from the body.

Failure of the blood supply to any part of the body naturally has serious consequences. In the brain for example it is likely to damage and even destroy the area affected and to cause paralysis of the part of the body which it controls. This is commonly the face, or an arm or a leg. Brain damage often comes on suddenly. When this happens the patient loses consciousness, at least for a time, and is said to have suffered a "stroke". Gradual failures of the blood supply more often affect other parts of the body such as the finger tips or toes, especially in old people. This causes a slow form of tissue damage known as gangrene, which can eventually involve the loss of the part affected.

The amounts of oxygen and nutrients, and therefore the amount of blood, needed by the tissues vary from moment to moment according to their state of activity. The most

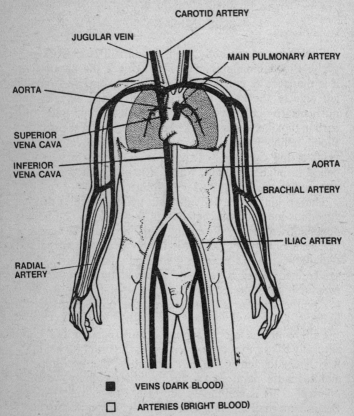

Fig. 1 The heart, the main arteries and veins. Note: pulmonary arteries show dark blood, see page 14.

striking examples are the muscles of the limbs and the muscles in the chest which are responsible for breathing. They need about five times as much blood during exercise as they do when the body is at rest.

THE CIRCULATION

The circulation is uniquely fitted to meet the changing needs of the body. Fig. 1 gives an overall view. There are three components, the blood which nourishes the tissues, the blood vessels which convey the blood to and from the tissues and the heart which pumps the blood.

Blood vessels are of three kinds, arteries, veins and capillaries. Arteries carry blood from the heart to the tissues and to the lungs, veins return blood from the tissues and lungs to the heart and capillaries connect the smallest arteries with the smallest veins. Fig. 2 clarifies this.

Two large arteries, the aorta and the pulmonary artery each with a diameter of about 3cm carry blood respectively from the left and right sides of the heart. The aorta, through its branches, takes blood to all parts of the body (the systemic circulation). The pulmonary artery takes blood to the lungs (the pulmonary circulation). See Fig. 3.

The systemic arteries originate in the aorta and divide into numerous branches to supply all parts of the body. They become smaller as their distance from the heart increases. In the tissues they narrow into capillaries which connect the smallest arteries with the smallest veins so that these can drain the tissues and then convey blood back to the right side of the heart.

The pulmonary artery divides into two main branches which take blood to the right and left lungs. Similarly their branches diminish in size until they join the pulmonary capillaries which in turn connect with the pulmonary veins which take blood back to the left heart. The complete circuit of the blood is thus from the left side of the heart out through the arteries to the body and back via the veins to the right heart, whence it is transmitted through the lungs before returning again to the left heart.

The purpose of the pulmonary circulation is to reoxygenate blood which has been deoxygenated by tissue activity. Deoxygenated blood is darker than oxygenated blood; consequently blood in the systemic veins, the right heart and the pulmonary arteries will be darker than that in the left heart, the systemic arteries and the pulmonary veins.

THE BLOOD VESSELS

Arteries are thick walled, elastic and muscular. Veins are thinner walled and less muscular. Their shape changes according to the amount of blood they contain. When full they are circular in cross section; when relatively empty they become flat and eliptical. The veins in the neck and the veins in the legs provide characteristic examples. When you stand up the veins in your legs are distended and circular to accommodate additional blood under the influence of gravity whilst the veins in your neck are flat and relatively empty. When you lie down the opposite happens. Capillaries are extremely numerous and very thin walled. Oxygen, nutrients and waste products cross their walls easily to enter or leave the tissues which they serve. Their total cross section is nearly 3000 times that of the aorta, but when the body is at rest only about a quarter of them are open. The remainder open when required to accommodate more blood.

The capacity of arteries and to a lesser extent of veins is determined by the degree of contraction of the muscles in their walls. These muscles are active to some extent all the time and so exert a degree of permanent control. The calibre of blood vessels controlled in this way is greatly influenced by chemical changes in the constitution of the blood brought about by changes in tissue metabolism. Arteries and veins, but not capillaries, are also under nervous control which will be described later. Suffice here to note that the process is complex but is an essential part of the

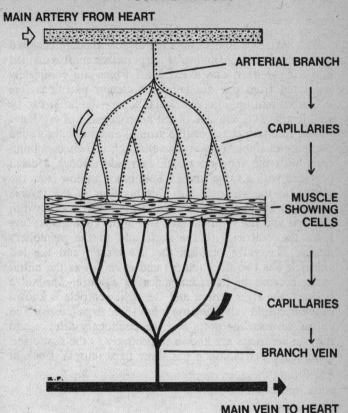

Fig. 2 Blood supply to and from muscle.

mechanism which maintains the circulation and enables it to adapt to the changing needs of the body. The size of the smallest arteries determines the resistance to blood flow in the circulation and is therefore important in controlling the blood pressure. The capacity of the veins controls the amount of blood returning to the heart and therefore influences the output of the heart.

THE HEART

The heart is a four chambered muscular pump enclosed in a membranous sac known as the pericardium. It is divided into a right heart and a left heart which are completely separated from one another by muscular partitions (the interatrial and the interventricular septa – the latter can be seen in Fig. 3). Each side of the heart consists of a thinner walled receiving chamber (the atrium) and a thicker walled pumping chamber (the ventricle). Each atrium communicates with the ventricle on its own side through a canal provided with a valve which allows blood to flow from the atrium to the ventricle but prevents flow in the reverse direction. There are four valves in the heart; two between the atria and the ventricles and two in the channels leading from the ventricles to the aorta and to the pulmonary artery. The valve between the left atrium and the left ventricle has two flaps (cusps) and is known as the mitral valve because of its resemblance to a mitre. The valve between the right atrium and the right ventricle is known as the tricuspid valve because it has three flaps (cusps). The valves between the aorta and the pulmonary arteries and the two ventricles are known respectively as the aortic and pulmonary valves. Each has three flaps (cusps). Look at Fig. 4.

How the heart works

The heart pumps the blood by alternately contracting and relaxing its muscular walls. Contraction (systole) reduces the size of a chamber, expels the blood from it and drives it onwards. Contraction of the left ventricle generates the driving force of the systemic circulation. In between beats the heart muscle relaxes (diastole) but the driving force is maintained sufficiently nevertheless to continue to propel blood into the right atrium through the veins pending the next beat. Two large veins enter the heart carrying this blood. The superior vena cava brings blood from all

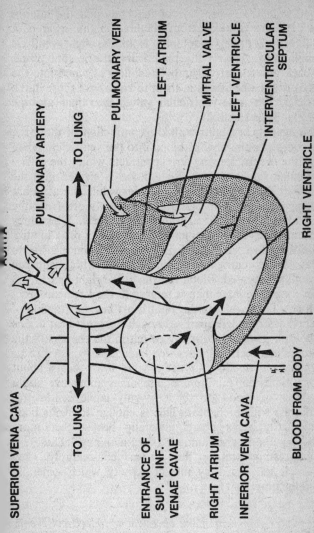

SUPERIOR VENA CAVA

PULMONARY ARTERY

TO LUNG

PULMONARY VEIN

LEFT ATRIUM

MITRAL VALVE

LEFT VENTRICLE

INTERVENTRICULAR SEPTUM

RIGHT VENTRICLE

TO LUNG

TO LUNG

ENTRANCE OF SUP. + INF. VENAE CAVAE

RIGHT ATRIUM

INFERIOR VENA CAVA

BLOOD FROM BODY

TRICUSPID VALVE

Fig. 3 Circulation in the heart. Dark arrows – used blood: White arrows – fresh blood.

the veins in the upper part of the body and the inferior vena cava brings blood from all those in the lower part. Similar force drives the blood from the right ventricle through the lungs, via the pulmonary arteries and veins, and back into the left atrium. The inflow of blood into the atria causes the pressures in them to rise above those in the ventricles. The atrio-ventricular valves then open and the ventricles begin to fill.

The heart beat begins with the contraction of the atria. This completes the flow of blood into the ventricles. When filled the ventricles in turn contract, while the atrio-ventricular valves close so that blood is ejected into the aorta and the pulmonary artery. Meanwhile the atria are relaxing again so that blood enters once more from the great veins and pulmonary vein respectively. When they have completed their contraction the ventricles relax in turn. While they do so the atrial pressure begins once again to rise above the ventricular pressure and the whole sequence of events is repeated. Blood returns to the right heart from the body a little later than it returns to the left heart from the lungs. Consequently the right heart beats a fraction of a second after the left heart. Although the heart beat begins in the atria it cannot normally be felt in the chest until the ventricles contract.

When you sit down quietly your heart beats about seventy times per minute and discharges about five and a half litres of blood or about seventy cubic centimetres (millilitres) with each beat. This is enough for your body at rest. Children's hearts generally beat rather more quickly, perhaps one hundred times a minute. These are average resting rates but they do vary considerably. They are much influenced by mental activity which generally makes the heart beat faster.

What makes your heart beat: chemical and electrical events

The heart muscle is composed of numerous muscle cells. Contraction of the heart is brought about by shortening of the individual muscle cells. This is caused by a chemical change within the cells which is activated by an electrical stimulus and is itself accompanied by electrical activity.

Each muscle cell is bounded by a membrane which is selectively permeable to electrolytes – that is to minerals in solution carrying an electrical charge. The electrolytes concerned are potassium, sodium and calcium each carrying a positive charge. When the heart muscle is relaxed in between beats the concentration of potassium is greater inside than outside the cell and the concentration of sodium is much greater outside the cell than inside it. This uneven concentration of electrolytes, particularly of potassium, creates a difference of electrical potential across the cell wall with the result that the interior of the cell is electrically negative in relation to the outside. The cell is then said to be polarised. On the principles of physics these uneven concentrations would tend to equalise by diffusion of electrolytes through the cell wall. But in the heart the tendency of potassium to flow outwards is counterbalanced by an opposing electrical force generated by the cell membrane. The tendency of sodium to flow inwards is opposed by chemical processes related to the metabolism of the cell. These are known as the "sodium pump".

The heart beat is brought about by repeated activation of the muscle cells by an electrical stimulus. This inactivates the sodium pump and increases the permeability of the cell membrane to sodium which then flows rapidly into the cell. The concentration of the electrolytes is thereby reversed and the interior of the cell becomes electrically positive in relation to the exterior. The cell is said to be "depolarised". Changes in the distribution of potassium and calcium also produce a flow of current but the sodium flux is responsible for the immediate overall change of electrical potential. The changed situation within the muscle cell after depolarisation once more reduces the permeability of the membrane to sodium. The "sodium pump" again becomes active and sodium is kept out of the cell whilst potassium re-enters it. The electrolytes resume their original distribution, the cell becomes "re-polarised" and is ready to be activated again!

Activation: the pacemaker and the conducting system

The stimulus to activation or depolarisation of the heart muscle is an electrical discharge arising in the "pacemaker". This is a node of specialised tissue (the sino-atrial node) situated at the back and upper (headward) part of the heart. The sino-atrial node depolarises and repolarises spontaneously and rhythmically although with a time sequence which differs from that of the heart. Depolarisation of the pacemaker sends a wave of electrical activity throughout the atria which depolarises them. The wave of activation then passes through another node situated between the atria and the ventricles (atrio-ventricular node) before travelling down a tract of conducting tissue which finally divides into two branches carrying the impulse through the ventricles (the atrio-ventricular bundle and the right and left bundle branches). In normal circumstances the atrio-ventricular node acts as a brake and slows the passage of the pacemaker's impulse. The electrical activity of the pacemaker is an essential process of life which begins early in foetal development.

The electrical consequences of activation: the electrocardiogram

Between beats all parts of the heart are at the same electrical potential. Consequently there is no flow of electrical current between them. Since activation (depolarisation) of the various parts of the heart occurs in sequence differences of electrical potential will arise on its surface during contraction. The surface of the activated or depolarised parts becomes electrically negative in relation to the surface of the inactive or polarised parts and as a result electrical current will flow from the depolarised to the polarised area. Because the chemical changes in the muscle cells are extremely rapid and because activation spreads quickly through the heart muscle the flow of current during the depolarisation will be abrupt in onset and brief in duration. Repolarisation occurring during relaxation follows a different pathway from depolarisation and occurs rather more slowly, but it still produces differences of potential and therefore a flow of current between different parts of the heart muscle.

The current flowing during both depolarisation and repolarisation is transmitted widely throughout the body and can be recorded by a Galvanometer connected to electrodes placed suitably on the body surface. A graphic record can be made of these events and it gives valuable information about the way in which the heart muscle is working. It is known as the Electrocardiogram and we shall look at some examples later in Chapters 3 and 6.

The blood supply of the heart

Like every other muscle the heart needs a rapidly adjustable blood supply. This is supplied by the coronary arteries. They are the first branches of the aorta and arise just beyond the aortic valves. There are two main arteries, a left and a right. The left coronary artery supplies the left side and the greater part of the front of the heart and the right coronary supplies the right side and much of the back of the heart, including usually the greater part of the conducting system. Shortly after its origin the left coronary artery divides into two main branches, a circumflex branch which runs round the left side of the heart supplying its upper border and part of the back and a descending branch which runs down between the two ventricles supplying each of them and the muscular partition between them (the inter-ventricular septum). The right coronary artery has no major branch but proceeds round the heart in a groove between the right atrium and the right ventricle.

Small communicating channels (anastomoses) exist between the terminal branches of the two coronary arteries.

When the coronary arteries are narrowed by obstructive disease the anastomoses tend to increase in size and thus help to protect areas of the heart served by damaged vessels. The coronary arteries terminate in capillaries. These join the coronary veins which enter the right atrium in a special pocket or sinus (the sinus venosus) and thus complete the coronary circulation.

The coronary circulation

The driving force of the coronary circulation is supplied by the mean pressure (i.e. the mean between systole and diastole, see page 16) in the aorta. However because the coronary arteries are embedded in the muscular walls of the heart they are squeezed when the muscle contracts and their resistance to flow is increased. Conversely they are released when the heart muscle relaxes and the resistance to blood flow is reduced. Coronary artery blood flow therefore differs from the blood flow in other arteries by being greater in between heart beats. Nervous activity increases coronary flow by its action on the heart beat. There is evidence of a direct action of the nervous system on the coronary arteries but nervous action on the heart itself probably has a greater influence on coronary flow.

BLOOD FLOW IN THE GENERAL BODY CIRCULATION

Subject to modifications caused by its complex character the circulation obeys the general principles governing the flow of fluid in a rigid tube. In such a system flow is proportional to the energy pressure within the system and inversely proportional to the resistance generated by the tube. This in turn is proportional to the length of the tube and inversely proportional to its cross section. In the circulation energy is intermittent and is provided by the contraction of the ventricles. Resistance is largely determined by the smaller arteries (arterioles) with their great total length and their diminishing cross section. Capillaries, and to a lesser extent veins make a smaller contribution.

Why the blood flows continuously between the heart beats

In a rigid tube system fluid flow is continuous only as long as the driving force is constant. If the driving force is intermittent flow will be intermittent. In the human circulation although the driving force of the heart beat is intermittent blood flow is continuous. You can yourself perform an experiment originally devised in the 17th Century which will explain how this happens. Place one end of a rubber tube with a valve at the other end, in water. Connect the valve end of this "inflow" tube to a rubber bulb which also has a rigid outflow tube. By alternately squeezing and relaxing the bulb you will suck water into the bulb through the inflow tube and then propel it into the outflow tube. It will emerge in a series of intermittent jets coinciding with the pressure generated by squeezing the bulb. If you replace the outflow tube with a narrower rigid tube the same will happen. Similarly, if you exchange the original rigid tube for an elastic one of that size the flow will still be in gulps. However, substitute an outflow tube which is both narrower *and* elastic, and flow will become continuous. In the circulation the aorta and the larger arteries are elastic, distending when the blood is ejected into them by the heart and recoiling in between each heart beat. This property together with the resistance set up by the smaller arteries (arterioles) ensures a continuous forward flow of blood in spite of the intermittent character of the heart beat.

Pressure and flow in the heart and circulation

The pressures in the heart and circulation are measured in millimetres of mercury (mm Hg.). The pressure in the left ventricle during contraction is about 130 mmHg. This enables it to eject blood into the aorta which has a pressure of about 70 mmHg. between each heart beat and which rises to about 120 mmHg. as blood is injected into it. Because of the resistance set up by the smaller arteries the blood pressure falls to about 30 mmHg. around the junction between them and the capillaries. A further fall occurs as the blood travels across the capillaries and reduces the pressure at their venous end to about 10 mmHg. This still exceeds the pressure in the right atrium which is around zero and together with assistance from contraction of the skeletal muscles ensures the return of blood to the heart. Some veins, especially those in the lower limbs, are provided with valves which prevent any flow of blood away from the heart while you are in the upright position. From the right atrium blood flows into the right ventricle. Flow begins when the pressure in the right atrium as it fills becomes equal to that in the ventricle as the latter relaxes after ejecting blood into the pulmonary artery. The filling of the ventricle thus is completed by the contraction of the atrium. Immediately afterwards the right ventricle begins to contract. This generates a pressure of about 25 mmHg. which is great enough to propel blood into the pulmonary artery with an average pressure of 16 mmHg., and onwards through the lungs into the pulmonary veins through which it returns to the left atrium where the pressure is about 6 mmHg. Pressures within the heart therefore vary during the different phases of the heart beat. They rise in each chamber when it contracts and fall when it relaxes. Pressures in the right heart are always lower than those in the left heart and the pressures in the atria are below those in the ventricles except when the latter are resting after ejecting their contents.

HOW THE HEART VALVES WORK

The heart valves open and close in response to changes in pressure on each side of them. The pressure changes just described should explain what they do and why they are important. When the atria are relaxed and admitting blood from the veins the tricuspid and mitral valves are closed because of the high pressure in the ventricles which

1 OPEN

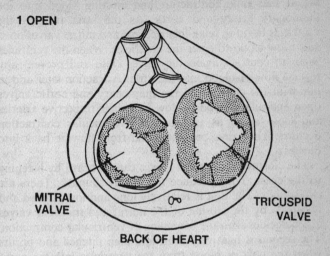

MITRAL
VALVE

TRICUSPID
VALVE

BACK OF HEART

2 CLOSED

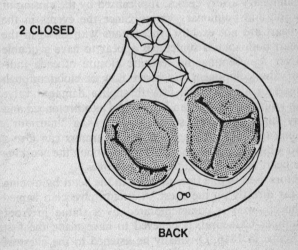

BACK

Fig. 4 Section showing heart valves.

are at that time contracting and ejecting blood into the pulmonary artery and aorta. As the atria fill and the ventricles begin to relax the tricuspid and mitral valves open and allow blood to enter the ventricles. When the ventricles begin to contract again the valves close and prevent any reverse flow of blood into the atria. A fraction later and in line with the contraction the pulmonary and aortic valves open and allow blood to flow into their respective arteries and close again as the force of ventricular contraction declines. They thus prevent blood from flowing back into the heart.

The closure of the heart valves can be heard by listening to the chest. They produce the "heart sounds". There are two sounds. The first is relatively long and low pitched and is caused by the closing of the mitral and tricuspid valves and coincides with the beginning of ventricular contraction. The second is relatively short and high pitched and occurs when the flow of blood from the ventricles into the aorta and pulmonary artery ceases. It is caused by the closing of the aortic and pulmonary valves. Since the events in the right heart are not exactly synchronous with those in the left heart both sounds sometimes appear to have a double character representing the separate closure of each individual valve component. Excessive flow of blood through the heart or an abnormal flow through a damaged valve sets up vibrations which can be detected as a prolonged and usually high frequency sound known as a "murmur". Listening to the heart sounds and to murmurs can give a trained observer valuable information about the working of the heart and the condition of the valves.

Doctors used at one time to listen to the heart by placing their ear directly on the chest. A Breton physician named "Laennec", who is commemorated by a statue in front of Quimper Cathedral, is believed to have made the first stethoscope in 1816. Originally he listened to the chest of a pregnant woman through his rolled up Medical Diploma. Afterwards single tube wooden stethoscopes were made and later increasingly sophisticated double rubber tubed stethoscopes which enabled physicians to listen with both ears and to pick up a greater range of sound frequencies.

The introduction of the stethoscope at the beginning of the 19th Century presented doctors with new and puzzling information which for some time caused much controversy about the nature of the heart sounds. A crucial experiment performed in 1830 by James Hope, a London physician, should have settled the matter. He opened the chest of a partially anaesthetised donkey and prevented the movements of each of the valves in turn by hooking them up with a bodkin whilst a colleague listened to the chest and noted the changes in the heart sounds. In spite of this convincing demonstration some years elapsed before the arguments finally ceased.

THE ARTERIAL PULSE

The pressure changes occurring in the aorta and in the main systemic arteries with each beat are transmitted along these vessels as a wave known as the arterial pulse. The height of the wave depends upon the difference between the pressure generated by each heart beat (the systolic pressure) and the pressure existing between the beats (the diastolic pressure). The speed at which the wave rises to its peak and the rate of its subsequent decline reflect changes in the rate and force with which the blood is ejected from the left ventricle into the aorta.

The arterial pulse is felt by placing a finger lightly on a convenient artery. It is most often used to determine the rate and the regularity of the heart beat. However it is also a rough and ready way of estimating its strength. A trained observer will find it equally useful in establishing the presence and in assessing the severity of valve disease. An obstructed aortic valve (aortic stenosis) for example produces a characteristic pulse which rises slowly to a plateau and then falls away gradually. An incompetent aortic valve, which allows blood to flow freely backwards into the ventricle when it is relaxing, produces a quick rising pulse wave which declines quickly – a "collapsing pulse". The artery at the wrist (the radial artery) is convenient and traditional for feeling the pulse but the artery at the bend of the elbow (the brachial artery) and the main artery in the neck (the carotid artery) are both larger and nearer to the heart and in certain circumstances give more accurate information. Disease of the larger arteries causing obstruction or partial obstruction to the flow of blood in them can sometimes be detected because it delays the arrival or reduces the volume of the pulse in the affected vessel.

Capillary pulsation

Very small arteries and capillaries do not pulsate unless they are dilated and unless the output of the heart is considerably increased and ejection into the aorta is forcible. Capillary pulsation causes alternate flushing and blanching of the skin in time with each heart beat, which can be best seen in the forehead or in the finger nails. It is found in conditions in which the output of the heart is persistently raised such as pregnancy and over-activity of the thyroid gland. It also occurs with incompetence of the aortic valve.

The arterial pressure: the venous pressure

Generally known as the blood pressure, the arterial pressure can be estimated in a medium sized artery such as the artery at the bend of the elbow (the brachial artery). This is generally done by compressing the artery externally by an inflatable cuff attached to a recording instrument (usually a mercury column) and by feeling the pulse below it. The pressure in the cuff is raised until the arterial pulse below the cuff disappears. The cuff is then released and the pressure at which the pulse reappears is taken as the systolic pressure. A fair indication of the systolic pressure can be obtained by feeling the pulse but it is more accurate to listen to the arterial pulse sounds with a stethoscope and to note the point at which they disappear as the cuff is inflated, and the point at which they return as the cuff is loosened again.

Listening also allows the diastolic pressure to be measured since the pulse sounds, returning as the cuff loosens, become louder and clearer until a point is reached when they disappear – usually abruptly. This marks the diastolic pressure. Pressures taken by this method are liable to be influenced by errors of observation and by the thickness of the subject's arm. Blood pressure is also influenced by tension and anxiety so that it should always be taken with the person as relaxed as possible, preferably lying down with a pillow or head rest. Three readings are usually made to ensure relaxation. Figures such as 135/90 mmHg., 125/85 mmHg. and 120/80 mmHg. can be recorded from successive readings in a normal person. Because of the limited accuracy of this method pressures are read to the nearest 1-2 mm/Hg.

The venous pulse

Large veins near the heart pulsate. This pulse, evident in the main veins in the neck (the jugular venous pulse), reflects the changes of pressure occurring in the right atrium during the heart beat. Because the pressure changes are small this pulse cannot be felt but it can usually be seen in the neck of a person sitting at an angle of about 40° from the horizontal. There are two peaks of higher pressure and two troughs of lower pressure. The first peak is caused by the rise of the pressure when the atrium contracts. The trough following it represents the relaxation of the atrium. The second peak which follows immediately afterwards occurs when the right ventricle contracts closing the tricuspid valve and interrupting the flow of blood from the atrium to the ventricle. The second trough occurs when the tricuspid valve opens again during ventricular relaxation and once more allows blood to flow from the atrium to the ventricle. Sometimes the first trough is interrupted by a small peak which is believed to be caused by the actual closure of the tricuspid valve. Changes of pressure in the left atrium are reflected similarly in the pulmonary veins. They cannot be seen directly but they can be recorded by cardiac catheterisation (see Chapter 6).

The central venous pressure

The pressures in the superior and inferior venae cavae are known as the central venous pressure, that is the pressure in the veins as they enter the heart. Central venous pressure is of great practical importance. It is influenced by several factors which include the total blood volume, the degree of "tone" in the vessel walls, the pressure in the right atrium, and the contraction of both the right atrium and of the right ventricle.

The central venous pressure can be measured accurately only by inserting a catheter into the superior or inferior venae cavae. In practice however it can be estimated from the vertical distance in centimetres (of blood) between the right atrium and the average height point of the venous pulse. As stated earlier the venous pulse can usually be seen in the main vein on the right side of the neck and is normally visible in a person sitting at 40° above the horizontal. If he sits up higher it disappears behind the collar bone; if he lies too flat it tends to disappear behind the angle of the jaw. Since the atrium itself cannot be seen the pressure is measured from the junction of the upper and lower parts of the breast bone (the sternal angle) which is nearly always 10 cm above the atrium. The vertical height of the pulse above this point should not exceed 3-4 cm. A venous pressure greater than this is abnormal and in the majority of cases is caused by increased pressure in the right atrium resulting from reduced efficiency of the heart. Another cause is obstruction to the flow of blood from the right ventricle by pulmonary valve disease. Incompetence of the tricuspid valve allows blood to flow backwards into the right atrium during ventricular contraction and sends a wave of high pressure back through the atrium and thence through the superior venae cavae and jugular veins. It may reach the angle of the jaw and is powerful enough to be mistaken sometimes for a pulse in an artery. Correct observation of the venous pulse is not easy and should be left to doctors who are trained to do it.

REGIONAL AND LOCAL BLOOD FLOW

The flow of blood to individual parts of the circulation generally depends on the state of the circulation as a whole but local variations are often necessary to meet particular demands in areas such as the brain, the kidneys, the heart itself, the muscles and the skin. The driving force of the heart is the same for all parts of the body at any given time. Changes in local flow therefore rely upon changes in the resistance set up by the smaller arteries serving the part in question. These depend either upon chemical changes in the blood resulting from increased tissue metabolism or upon alterations in nervous control. Chemical changes are generally more important particularly in the brain, the heart and the muscles. Of these oxygen lack, carbon dioxide excess and increased acid production are the most significant. Oxygen lack and carbon dioxide excess both dilate arteries and so increase tissue blood flow. Acids and other waste products probably have a similar effect but it is not clear how they act and which of them is particularly important. Nervous control is particularly important in the skin, but arteries there are also affected by changes in temperature, being narrowed by cold and enlarged by heat.

THE NERVOUS CONTROL OF THE HEART AND CIRCULATION

As stated earlier the heart and the blood vessels, apart from the capillaries, are under the influence of the nervous system. The part concerned is the sympathetic or "autonomic" system as it is sometimes called because it functions independently of conscious control. The autonomic system includes both sympathetic and parasympathetic nerves. These nerves act by releasing chemical substances at the point where they terminate in the tissues. Parasympathetic nerves release acetylcholine. Sympathetic nerves generally release adrenaline and noradrenaline although some sympathetic nerves found in muscle release acetylcholine.

Sympathetic nerves quicken the heart beat and increase its force. They also affect the blood vessels. They are particularly numerous in the smaller arteries which supply the resistance to the circulation and in the smaller veins which regulate the capacity of the veins to hold blood. Their action is generally to narrow (constrict) both arteries and veins and thus to increase the resistance to blood flow in the arteries and decrease the capacity of the veins to hold blood.

Parasympathetic nerves have their most important action on the heart. They slow its rate and decrease the force of atrial contraction, and thus indirectly the force of the heart beat. They are also found in blood vessels but their overall effect, which is to enlarge the vessels, is small in comparison with the ability of the sympathetic nerves to constrict.

The regulation of the circulation and the maintenance of a steady blood pressure depend to a certain extent upon the balance between sympathetic and parasympathetic nervous activity. Under ordinary conditions when lying down the heart is under "tonic control" of the parasympathetic nerves but the sympathetic system will come into action to enable it to meet extra demands e.g. on standing up. The smaller arteries and veins are as a rule under mild tonic control of the sympathetic nerves.

The nervous control of the heart and blood vessels is regulated by a complex process depending largely upon reflex activity. A centre situated in the lower part of the brain (the medulla) discharges regular impulses through the sympathetic nerves. The rate of discharge is regulated by signals transmitted by incoming nerves connected to receptor points in the tissues which they supply. These circulatory receptors are situated in the walls of the aorta, in the main artery to the brain (the carotid artery), in the superior and the inferior venae cavae and in the pulmonary veins where they join the heart. They are also present in the pulmonary arteries and in the heart itself. They are sensitive to stretching of the vessels where they are situated and thus indirectly to changes in pressure and volume. Increased stretch, caused by increased pressure, increases the number of impulses going to the brain centre which responds by reducing the number of outgoing sympathetic impulses. Consequently the heart slows, the resistance in the circulation is decreased and the blood pressure tends to fall. Conversely decreased stretch associated with a fall in pressure in the main blood vessels provokes increased central activity which raises the rate and force of the heart beat and narrows the resistance vessels and the smaller veins and so tends to increase the blood pressure and the return of the blood to the heart. This compensatory mechanism is particularly important when there is a sudden fall of blood pressure such as happens with severe loss of blood or by a sudden reduction of the heart's output such as occurs with a coronary attack. (See explanations).

The nervous control of the heart and circulation is also affected by chemical changes in the blood. They are "picked up" by a receptor in the artery to the brain (the carotid artery), which is sensitive to oxygen lack and to changes in blood acidity. Oxygen lack and increased acidity resulting from increased tissue metabolism reduces the ingoing signals to the brain centre in a manner similar to that of changes of pressure and with comparable effects. Apart from these reflex effects the brain centre also responds to impulses generated in the higher parts of the brain as a result of mental activity and emotion and changes in body temperature.

HOW THE HEART MEETS DEMAND FOR EXTRA BLOOD DURING EXERCISE

The heart meets demands for extra blood during exercise by increasing its rate and by increasing its output per beat (stroke volume). The relative importance of each of these two processes is difficult to determine and may vary with the nature of the demand. Trained athletes, for example, probably differ slightly from untrained people in the way in which they respond to the demands of strenuous exercise.

The increased heart rate during exercise is the result of increased sympathetic nerve activity which is partly central and partly reflex in origin. The increased stroke volume is partly the result of increased sympathetic activity provoked in a number of ways and partly the result of an increased volume of blood being returned to the heart. This is the result of decreased resistance in the smaller arteries which increases the blood flow into the veins. It is greatly assisted by the squeezing action of the exercising muscles on the veins themselves. This increased return of blood stretches the heart muscle and makes it contract more forcibly. These two processes working together can raise the heart's output of blood very quickly from about five to twenty-five litres a minute.

Nervous influences and chemical changes in the contracting muscles also influence local blood flow. Initially a discharge of acetylcholine by sympathetic nerves probably causes dilatation of arteries in the exercising muscles and helps to increase their blood supply. Later chemical changes associated with the increased muscular activity continue the process. Generally at the start of exercise the increased output of the heart causes the blood pressure to rise but with enlargement (dilatation) of the resistance arteries it tends to fall again. As the exercise continues a steady level not greatly above normal is reached. Static muscular effort (isometric contraction) such as when lifting a heavy weight or pushing a stationary car raises the heart rate without dilating the smaller arteries and causes a sharp increase in blood pressure, which continues until the exertion ceases.

THE CIRCULATION DURING PREGNANCY

The essential feature of the circulation in pregnancy is that the blood volume is increased. The increase begins during the second month and has become substantial by the end of the third month. Subsequently a further gradual increase takes place until by the thirty-second week, there is an increase of up to 45% above the normal. Thereafter the blood volume remains steady. The increase is the result partly of increased retention of salt and water in the body and partly of circulatory changes occurring in the womb. The increased bood volume causes an increased return of blood to the heart and an associated increase of about a half in the heart's output (high output state). The heart consequently becomes slightly enlarged and beats forcibly with a moderate increase in rate. The feet and hands tend to become hot and the face flushed. The smaller arteries pulsate vigorously and pulsation in the capillaries can sometimes be detected by alternate blanching and flushing of the skin which can best be seen in the forehead and the beds of the finger nails when they are gently compressed.

The blood pressure in pregnancy

The increased output of the heart tends to raise the blood pressure but normally it is counterbalanced by the lowered resistance in the circulation because of enlargement (dilatation) of the smaller arteries. In fact the systolic pressure usually falls slightly and the diastolic pressure falls appreciably. Occasionally, probably in those with a constitutional tendency towards high blood pressure, high blood pressure develops in mid pregnancy but returns to normal after the birth of the child. Sometimes it persists. Severe rises of pressure with signs of kidney damage (toxemia) are abnormal and need expert management.

Prospects for pregnancy with heart disease

The additional circulatory demands of pregnancy do not trouble the healthy heart but carry risks for those with heart disease. Modern methods of treatment however including for example emergency operations on valves, have considerably improved the outlook and most women with heart disease can nowadays look forward to having one or even more than one child safely. But where heart trouble is present careful medical supervision throughout pregnancy is imperative. The chief hazard during pregnancy used to be valvular disease of rheumatic origin. This still exists particularly in developing countries but is becoming rarer. Heart disease caused by high blood pressure, by congenital abnormalities and heart muscle disease from a variety of causes can also be encountered. With heart disease the chief risk to mothers is the liability to develop some degree of heart failure (see Chapter 3) from the third month onwards. Both labour and the period immediately after birth (the Puerperium) are the periods of greater danger. Termination of pregnancy for this reason is still sometimes necessary when life is threatened. To be effective it should be undertaken in the early months.

2
THE NATURE OF
HEART DISEASE

Broadly speaking there are five ways in which disease affects the heart. They are disease of the heart muscle, disease of the conducting system, disease caused by abnormal loads on the heart, valvular disease and congenital malformation. Disease can also affect the pericardium. Minor degrees of heart disease often cause no trouble at all and even serious disease can be present for long periods, perhaps for years, without making the heart go wrong. This chapter discusses mainly the nature of heart disease. The ways in which the diseased heart *goes wrong* are discussed in the next chapter.

HEART MUSCLE DISEASE

Disease affecting the heart muscle may be acute – in the sense that it produces its effects rapidly and then subsides fairly quickly – or it may be chronic with gradual and protected effects.

Communicable diseases provide characteristic examples of acute heart muscle disease. Inflammation by bacteria such as streptococci and staphylococci, and by mycoplasma (see explanations) is usually a sequel to a generalised infection starting in the throat, the skin or other soft tissues, or in the lungs. Virus disease is always difficult to identify but heart disease has been clearly associated with influenza and with a group of viruses capable of causing generalised muscle disease named Coxsackie viruses. The group was named after the place in the United States where it was first discovered.

Two important acute diseases of bacterial origin are Rheumatic Fever and Diphtheria. Both still exist, particularly in developing countries but are becoming rarer elsewhere because of increasingly effective means of prevention. Rheumatic Fever which was once responsible for about a third of all heart disease is an allergic reaction to infection by a particular strain of streptococcus. Fever can be severe and many parts of the body, notably the larger joints are likely to be involved. The most serious and lasting effects which may occur are on the heart. The disease attacks not only the heart muscle and the pericardium but also the valves, where it not infrequently causes severe and permanent damage. This is discussed later. Occasionally the muscle damage is severe and can lead to a degree of heart failure. The greatest incidence of Rheumatic Fever is in children and teenagers. Characteristically it occurs in attacks, preceded usually by a sore throat. They last for about six weeks but have a tendency to recur over a period of years. Diphtheria is even less common nowadays because of immunisation in childhood. It is a bacterial infection which starts in the throat and causes chemical (toxic) damage to nerves as well as to the heart muscle. The conducting system is also particularly likely to be affected. Occasionally sudden death can occur during the acute illness, but as a rule the heart recovers completely after a period of weeks or months.

The heart muscle can also be damaged by infestation by parasites such as toxoplasma in temperate climates and trypanosomes (see explanation) in the tropics. An uncommon but serious cause of acute damage to the heart muscle is accidental or sometimes suicidal poisoning by carbon monoxide.

Generalised diseases causing more chronic damage include severe anaemia and severe nutritional deficiencies, particularly of Vitamin B. Disease of the thyroid gland, whether showing increased activity (Thyrotoxicosis – Graves Disease) or diminished activity (Myxoedema) characteristically affect the heart muscle. Thyrotoxicosis

when severe and untreated is particularly likely to lead to a
measure of heart failure and in older subjects to disorders
of the heart beat, notably atrial fibrillation (see Chapter 3).
Myxoedema which is the result of grossly deficient thyroid
activity has profound effects on many parts of the body
and is liable to cause severe damage to the heart muscle.
Treatment with thyroid gland extract or one of its components is effective but can aggravate the heart trouble
unless it is very carefully controlled. Rarer diseases affecting
the heart are familial (genetic) disorders both of the muscle
and of the nervous system. Successful treatment of some
causal diseases described can generally bring about a
complete recovery in the heart.

Muscle disease – confined mainly to the heart

Muscle disease is sometimes apparently confined to the
heart. Disease of this kind includes a rather infrequent kind
of heart muscle disease for which there is no generally
accepted cause. It is known as cardiomyopathy. A family
history occasionally suggests a genetic abnormality but
more often the disease occurs without any of the more usual
known causes.

Cardiomyopathy is mostly discovered because it has led
to some degree of heart failure (see Chapter 3), breathlessness on exertion, or occasionally pain characteristic of
Angina Pectoris (see next section). Sometimes it is detected
in apparently healthy people – where it can cause sudden
death – only by a chance medical examination. Cardiomyopathy generally only begins to cause trouble in early
adult life and may not appear before middle age.

Opinions differ about the capacity of alcohol to produce
heart muscle disease. Impurities in alcoholic drinks such
as cobalt in beer have been implicated but very rarely.
Alcohol itself can cause a deficiency of Vitamin B giving
rise to Beri Beri, a disease causing heart muscle damage
which is otherwise almost exclusively confined to tropical
countries. However there is little doubt that prolonged and

heavy consumption of alcohol directly damages the heart muscle and can lead in time to serious heart failure. Only too often the disease is in an advanced stage before it is detected. Treatment is correspondingly disappointing but cure is possible if alcohol is given up before serious damage has occurred.

Heart muscle disease as a side effect caused by other illness is often overlooked. Usually it recovers, probably completely, once the causal condition has subsided or been controlled by treatment. Sometimes however disorders of the heart beat are provoked or, when the illness has been severe as in Rheumatic Fever or Alcoholic muscle disease, a degree of heart failure may arise. Even so the heart can recover if treatment is undertaken as soon as the illness is recognised.

The main danger in milder cases is that no thought is given to possible heart disease.

Strenuous physical exertion in the circumstances can be dangerous. For example athletes resuming training before they have fully recovered from some relatively mild fever have died suddenly, probably because of the sudden onset of a serious disorder of the heart beat.

Coronary artery disease

By far the commonest cause of heart muscle disease is coronary artery disease. Healthy coronary arteries supply the heart with enough blood and hence nutrition to enable it to maintain an effective circulation under all conditions. Disease damages the arteries and impairs their ability to supply blood. This in turn damages the heart muscle and limits its capacity to respond to the demands of physical exertion. Exercise becomes liable to provoke characteristic pain and discomfort in the chest (Angina Pectoris), described from page 87. Complete obstruction of a coronary artery or one of its branches deprives part of the heart muscle of its blood supply causing acute damage to the affected area. It is responsible for the clinical condition known as Coronary

Thrombosis or more popularly as a "Coronary". This is because the obstruction is usually caused by thrombosis (see page 77). Coronary Heart Disease is discussed in detail in Chapter 4.

DAMAGE TO THE CONDUCTING SYSTEM

Disease of the heart muscle, particularly inflammatory disease and Diptheria sometimes involves the conducting system. Drugs such as digitalis used in the treatment of heart failure (see page 65), adrenaline antagonists such as propranolol, and antimony preparations sometimes used in the treatment of tropical diseases all have possible effects which doctors must take into account when using them. Damage to the conducting system caused by agents of this kind is usually transient and is likely to recover when the cause is removed. Permanent damage is sometimes the result of coronary artery disease but more often of a specific· destructive disease of uncertain origin. The effects of disease of the conducting system vary according to the severity of the damage but in general they consist of a lesser or greater degree of heart block. This is described in Chapter 3.

DAMAGE TO THE HEART BY ABNORMAL LOADS IN THE CIRCULATION

High blood pressure: (Pulmonary hypertension)

The healthy heart meets the normal demands of the circulation without difficulty. Exceptional but intermittent demands such as those of prolonged physical exertion, as in marathon running, may cause some hypertrophy or thickening of the heart muscle just as may occur in other muscles with prolonged use. Provided that it is healthy, the heart is undamaged and its efficiency is unimpaired. A healthy heart may even maintain a prolonged persistently high output safely, as it may have to in pregnancy and for a time in anaemia. However, abnormally high pressures in the circulation, if they last long enough, nearly always impose a strain on the heart which leads to changes in the muscle and ultimately to weakness and some degree of heart failure.

High Blood Pressure (discussed fully in Chapter 5) raises the pressure in the systemic circulation causing hypertrophy and ultimately failure of the left ventricular muscle. High pressure in the pulmonary circulation (pulmonary hypertension) similarly affects the right ventricle. There are a number of causes. It can occur apparently by itself and without obvious cause but it is more often secondary either to longstanding disease of the left heart, particularly mitral stenosis as explained under its own heading on page 45, or to chronic lung diseases such as bronchitis and emphysema (see explanations). Another important cause is obstruction of the pulmonary artery and its branches by repeated embolism or local thrombosis. The precise medical meaning of these terms can be found in the explanations at the back. Obstruction of the main pulmonary artery or one of its branches by a thrombus (clot) which has become detached from its site of origin in a deep vein (usually in the lower abdomen or the lower limbs) is serious and dangerous. It is liable to occur in people who have been confined to bed by illnesses such as coronary thrombosis or in old people after fractures of the hip or after a surgical operation, particularly an abdominal operation. It can produce a sudden and severe rise in pulmonary artery pressure which can be fatal because of failure of the right heart. A number of methods designed to prevent its occurrence in people at risk have been tried with encouraging prospects. They include the use of drugs capable of interfering with the clotting processes of the blood as well as physical measures such as exercises in bed and getting up as soon as possible after operations and severe illness.

VALVULAR DISEASE AND CONGENITAL MALFORMATION

The effects of valvular disease and congenital malformation are in some ways similar since both interfere with the flow of blood within the heart. For instance, a congenital communication between the left and right heart (there should be none) such as a hole in the heart can lead to excess of blood in one or more chambers which then becomes overfilled and enlarged (dilated). A similar overfilling arises after a valve which has become ineffective because of disease allows blood to flow backwards into a chamber from which it has just been ejected preventing it being empty in readiness to receive its next quota of blood. Imperfect development of one of the great arteries leaving the heart (the aorta or the pulmonary artery) and narrowing of a valve by disease (stenosis) both tend to obstruct the onward flow of blood from the appropriate chamber. In each case the pressure in the chamber affected rises and the chamber itself tends to enlarge. Thickening (hypertrophy) of its muscular wall generally follows and enables it to contract more powerfully in an attempt to overcome the disability. The extent and effectiveness of this so called compensatory hypertrophy depend on the chambers involved and upon whether they are healthy or damaged by disease. Provided that they are not damaged by disease and that they have an adequate blood supply, the ventricles hypertrophy more effectively than the atria and they can often maintain the circulation almost normally for a time. Eventually however hypertrophied muscle outgrows its blood supply and weakens so that in due course the heart begins to fail.

VALVULAR DISEASE

Valvular disease, other than isolated pulmonary valve disease which is nearly always congenital, is usually acquired after birth and affects the valves in the left side of the heart (the mitral and aortic valves) more often than those on the right. Both the mitral and the tricuspid valves may also be stretched by dilatation of either the left or right ventricles respectively caused by disease. Though healthy in themselves they may be unable to function properly.

The commonest causes of valve damage used to be Rheumatic Fever which damages the mitral and the aortic valves, but particularly the mitral, and Syphilis which damages the aortic valve. Both diseases are nowadays better controlled. Consequently valvular disease is less common and is more likely to be the result of ageing in the case of the mitral valve or based on a congenital abnormality where there is aortic valve disease. Coronary thrombosis may also damage the mitral valve. Rheumatic Fever damages valves by inflammation during the active phase of the disease. At first they become swollen and unable to close properly but they may recover completely. More often scarring occurs especially where there have been recurrent attacks of the disease and the affected valves become distorted and stiffened and lose their mobility. Sometimes the valve flaps

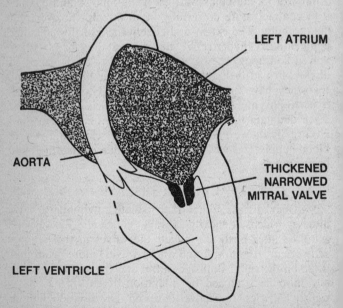

LEFT ATRIUM

AORTA

THICKENED NARROWED MITRAL VALVE

LEFT VENTRICLE

Fig. 5 Narrowing (stenosis) of mitral valve with enlargement of left atrium from increased pressure.

(cusps) become fused together causing narrowing of the channel which they control and so obstructing the flow of blood. Alternatively they may be bound down and so distorted that they fail to close properly and this allows blood to regurgitate against the normal direction of flow. The first situation is known as stenosis (narrowing) and the second as incompetence. Though stenosis and incompetence usually occur separately they may be present together causing the damaged valve to be both narrow and incompetent. Both conditions impose a strain on the heart muscle which is generally progressive.

Despite so many fewer cases of Rheumatic Fever occurring in recent years there are still a fair number of people needing treatment for Rheumatic Valvular Disease. This is because there is usually a long interval between the initial infection of the valve and the onset of symptoms caused by its effect on the heart. Also fresh cases of Rheumatic Fever continue to occur, especially in developing countries.

Narrowed Valves (*Mitral and Aortic Stenosis*)

Narrowing of a valve obstructs the onward flow of blood and tends to raise the pressure in the obstructed chamber accordingly. Minor degrees may have little effect but in the long run any significant such rise of pressure increases the work of the heart muscle and leads either to hypertrophy of it or dilatation (see explanations) or to both.

Mitral stenosis obstructs the flow of blood from the left atrium to the left ventricle. Look at Fig. 5. Small amounts of stenosis have little serious effect and allow the heart to function normally. Greater degrees of narrowing force the left atrium to generate a higher pressure of contraction than normal in order to overcome the obstruction and to maintain the flow of blood into the left ventricle. The greater pressure in the left atrium in turn causes a rise of pressure in the pulmonary veins and in due course in the pulmonary arteries and in the right ventricle. All affected chambers hypertrophy in an attempt to cope with the increased work but in spite of this the pressure in the left atrium continues to increase gradually. The situation is often aggravated by active constriction of the pulmonary arteries which further increases the pulmonary artery pressure and the strain on the right heart. However this arterial constriction also increases the resistance to flow in the pulmonary circulation and so to some extent protects the lungs.

The course of mitral stenosis is generally protracted. In the first place narrowing of the valve develops only gradually often following repeated attacks of inflammation. Secondly the compensatory measures described help to maintain the heart's function almost normally for some time. Even with severe narrowing an interval of years may elapse before the disease causes serious disability. In due course however except where the damage is trivial the heart begins to fail. In this situation exceptional demands upon the circulation such as occur during pregnancy or during some generalised infection sometimes precipitate a severe rise of pressure in the pulmonary veins. The lungs can become almost waterlogged and the patient dangerously breathless. More often however, unless the disease is treated (usually surgically) there is a gradual deterioration with increasing limitation of activity. At some stage a disorder of the heart beat such as atrial fibrillation (see Chapter 3) is to be expected. Medical and sometimes surgical treatment is then necessary.

Aortic stenosis obstructs the passage of blood from the left ventricle into the aorta. Though sometimes rheumatic it is more often based upon a congenitally abnormal valve which has only two (bicuspid) or rarely one leaflet (cusp) instead of the usual three. The degree of obstruction is usually progressive over a period of years because thrombosis and calcification (see explanations) take place in the valve. At first, the left ventricle hypertrophies without enlarging its chamber and copes well enough to protect the circulation but the patient's capacity for exertion becomes gradually more limited. Eventually the left ventricle weakens and the heart may begin to fail.

This can happen suddenly with cardiac asthma (see Chapter 3). Attacks of faintness or of anginal pain (see Chapter 4) are likely with aortic stenosis, especially on exertion, when the obstructed valve prevents the heart from meeting the needs of the brain a nd of the coronary circulation adequately at times of additional demand. The course of the disease is variable but it may last until the age of 50 or 60 before the onset of serious symptoms. Sudden death sometimes occurs.

Incompetent valves (Mitral and Aortic incompetence – Tricuspid incompetence – Pulmonary incompetence)

Incompetent valves allow blood to flow backwards into the chamber from which it has just been ejected.

Mitral incompetence allows blood to regurgitate from the left ventricle to the left atrium with each ventricular contraction. The left atrium which also receives blood from the lungs at the same time as the regurgitated blood, becomes overfilled. More blood is then discharged into the left ventricle which in turn becomes overfilled and discharges a greater volume of blood. (Some of it once again flows back into the left atrium.) In this situation both the left atrium and the left ventricle become dilated and hypertrophied. In the absence of obstruction at the mitral valve the pressure in the left atrium is however lower than in mitral stenosis and the pulmonary circulation is therefore less affected. Generally the heart's function is well maintained, often for some years, depending on the severity of the valvular leak. When the heart's function eventually does deteriorate it is liable to do so fairly rapidly.

Aortic Incompetence allows blood to regurgitate from the aorta into the left ventricle when it is relaxing in readiness to receive its normal quota of blood from the left atrium. The left ventricle becomes overfilled and has to do more work. Dilatation and hypertrophy follow but a remarkably efficient circulation can be maintained, sometimes for a long time. Minor degrees of damage can permit considerable physical exertion and even a fair level of athletic performance. Failure of the left ventricle, sometimes of rapid onset with cardiac asthma (see page 68), is eventually likely in severe cases but even moderately severe aortic incompetence may be symptomless until well into middle life. Accidents such as rupture of the damaged valve, possibly following strenuous exercise, can complicate the natural course of the disease.

Tricuspid incompetence is nearly always caused by stretching of the valve as a result of considerable enlargement of the right ventricle and not by direct disease of the valve. It is nearly always the result of a continued rise in pulmonary artery pressure and is characteristically found in association with Mitral Stenosis. In tricuspid incompetence both the right atrium and the right ventricle are enlarged and blood regurgitates from the ventricle to the atrium during each ventricular contraction. This causes a wave of pressure to travel through the atrium on into the great veins. It can be seen in the deep veins of the neck where it causes a powerful pulse occurring with each ventricular contraction and often extending as far as the angle of the jaw or even higher. By itself tricuspid incompetence causes little extra disability and it is chiefly important as a sign of severe and usually longstanding disease of the right heart.

Pulmonary incompetence is generally of secondary importance. It usually occurs either when the pulmonary valve is also stenosed or when the pulmonary artery is enlarged because of an extra large volume of blood being circulated to the lungs such as occurs with atrial septal defect (see page 54).

Bacterial Endocarditis (*valves infected by bacteria*)

Although Valvular Disease is often the result of inflammation which is, as in Rheumatic Fever, of bacterial origin bacteria are not usually found on the valves themselves. Bacterial endocarditis means that the valves are directly infected by bacteria. The severity of the disease depends largely on the way it has arisen.

Organisms particularly responsible are staphylococci, often arising in a wound, streptococci starting in the throat or in the skin, and pneumococci associated with infections of the lungs. Blood stream infection by these organisms may affect a number of organs in the body. It can cause severe damage to the heart and valves, usually either the aortic or mitral valve. Rarely an acute form (septicaemia) can occur during the course of any severe bacterial infection where disease producing organisms are circulating in the blood. Acute bacterial endocarditis is a dangerous complication of a serious illness. The heart muscle as well as the valves is likely to be affected and the combined damage is only too likely to lead to intractable and fatal heart failure. Fortunately the incidence of this disease has become rarer since the introduction of antibiotics for the treatment of acute infection.

Subacute bacterial endocarditis is commoner and is caused by infection of the blood by relatively less damaging organisms and especially by a strain of streptococcus (streptococcus viridans) which produces a greenish colour when cultivated on a medium containing blood. This organism is a common inhabitant of the mouth and often gains access to the blood at the time of dental extraction. The valves affected are nearly always abnormal due to previously existing, although generally symptomless, disease. Congenital abnormalities such as a hole between the ventricles or a patent ductus arteriosus (see page 56) may also be the site of the disease. "Vegetations" consisting of an infected thrombus (see explanations) form on the damaged valve. Clinically the disease has two characteristic features, a low grade but persistent fever and a tendency to embolism formation. Embolism means the blockage of an artery by some obstructing agent such as a part of a thrombus which has been carried from a distant site in the circulation. In the case of bacterial endocarditis it comes from a heart valve. The area of the body supplied by the blocked artery is suddenly, and sometimes permanently, deprived or partly deprived of its blood supply with the usual result: immediate and sometimes permanent loss of function.

Embolism in subacute bacterial endocarditis occurs repeatedly and may attack almost any organ of the body, the most important being the brain, the kidneys and spleen, the lungs and the skin. Brain embolism causes a stroke, often associated initially with loss of consciousness and with the sudden onset of a greater or lesser degree of paralysis. Embolism in the lungs causes pain in the chest and spitting of blood. Embolism in the kidneys causes pain in the loin and the passage of blood in the urine and in the spleen it causes pain under the left lower ribs. Embolism in the skin causes pain with localised areas of swelling and tenderness and sometimes haemorrhages in the nail beds.

Persons known to have a valve abnormality can usually be protected against Bacterial Endocarditis by the use of suitable antibiotics particularly before tooth extraction. Once detected the disease must be treated actively with suitable antibiotics, otherwise it can be fatal in a matter of weeks or months. The diagnosis is often difficult but signs of low grade infection in the presence of valvular disease or of a congenital abnormality justify immediate treatment (see pages 58 and 132).

CONGENITAL MALFORMATION

How the heart is formed before birth

The development of the heart in the womb is complex. Basically it involves the conversion of a straight tube with a venous and an arterial end into a four chambered heart with the venous end joined to the great veins from the body and the lungs and the arterial end merged into the arteries to the lungs (the pulmonary arteries) and into the artery to the remainder of the body (the aorta). Development occurs chiefly during the first three months of pregnancy with a critical period between the fifth and eighth week. By the fourth week of life in the womb the foetal heart begins to beat.

The foetal circulation

The essential difference between the foetal and the normal circulation is that the lungs which oxygenate the blood after birth are unable to do so in the womb. Blood has to be oxygenated in another way. This is done by the placenta (later to become the afterbirth). It receives deoxygenated blood from the foetus in the arteries of the umbillical cord and returns relatively oxygenated blood to it via the umbillical veins. This partially oxygenated blood eventually enters the right heart of the foetus in the inferior vena cava. The greater part is then transferred directly to the left heart through a communication between the right atrium and the left atrium (the foramen ovale) and is then circulated to different parts of the body through the aorta and its major branches. The remainder of the blood in the right heart circulates partly to the lungs but most of it reaches the aorta through a short communicating channel between that vessel and the main pulmonary artery (the ductus arteriosus). Blood from the lower branches of the aorta is returned in the umbillical arteries to the placenta. By this means all parts of the foetus receive blood which is oxygenated but at a lower level of saturation than adult blood. When breathing begins at birth the lungs expand and take in air and the blood flowing through them is oxygenated. Shortly afterwards the resistance and the pressure in the pulmonary arteries, which in the womb were higher than those in the systemic arteries, fall, the foramen ovale and the ductus arteriosus close, and effective blood flow through the lungs completes the change to a normal circulation.

Incidence of congenital malformations

Between three and four out of every thousand infants born alive are likely to have some congenital abnormality of the heart or of the great vessels. Such abnormalities have been estimated to account for about two per cent of all cases of heart disease. Practically every part of the heart as well as the adjoining parts of the great vessels can be affected. Some malformations are incompatible with sustained life outside the womb. A brief account of this kind can describe only the commoner defects occurring in clinical practice.

The origin of congenital malformations

Some congenital malformations are thought to be genetic in origin but the majority seem to be the result of the mother catching an infection or possibly suffering some at present unidentified metabolic upset during the first three months of pregnancy. The most firmly established cause is German Measles but infections by viruses such as the coxsackie virus and other viruses including influenza are increasingly recognised as responsible. The majority of congenital malformations arise from a faulty development of the primitive heart or its blood vessels. The most serious malformations arise in the first three months of pregnancy but failure to adapt to the circulatory changes occurring after birth is responsible for one major and one lesser abnormality. Direct infection of the heart occurring in the womb when the heart is almost fully developed probably causes foetal valvular disease.

The chief developmental abnormalities are faulty development of the partitions (septa) which separate the right heart from the left, faulty development of the arterial end of the primitive heart into the pulmonary artery and the aorta, and failure to develop the valve controlled channels which separate the atria from the ventricles. Failure to adapt to the circulatory changes occurring at birth leads to persistence of the foramen ovale and also to continued patency (openness) of the ductus arteriosus.

Congenital abnormalities may be single but often occur in combination particularly when development has been severely affected at the critical period (the fifth to eighth week of life in the womb). Some malformations such as an isolated patent foramen ovale are of little consequence but the majority impose strains upon the heart muscle which sooner or later lead to a measure of heart failure unless corrected surgically.

Blue babies

A characteristic manifestation of certain types of congenital heart disease is the so called blue baby. A number of different malformations may be responsible but the basic disorder common to all of them is that unoxygenated blood is directly shunted from the right heart to the left heart without going through the lungs. It is then circulated through the body. This gives the baby the bluish colour known as cyanosis (blueness). Its intensity depends upon the amount of unoxygenated blood circulated in this way. With small amounts the blue colour can be almost imperceptible and sometimes appears intermittently; with greater amounts it becomes intense and persistent. It is most easily seen in the face and lips but all visible parts of the body are affected. It is also seen in the inside of the mouth and under the tongue. This distinguishes it from "peripheral" cyanosis (see explanations). The body attempts to compensate for the inadequate oxygenation of the blood in "central" cyanosis by increasing the production of red blood cells. This in itself sometimes leads to trouble because arteries and veins can occasionally be blocked by thrombus formation (see Chapter 4) with serious local consequences. The severely cyanosed blue baby has an intense purplish blue colour often accompanied by swelling of the nail beds in the fingers and toes leading to a condition known as "clubbing". Growth may be stunted although mental development is usually normal. Physical activity can be greatly limited by breathlessness and affected children often squat frequently because the squatting position seems to help their breathing.

Holes in the heart – (ventricular and atrial septal defects)

A hole between the ventricles (ventricular septal defect) is the result of incomplete development of the muscular partition separating the left from the right ventricle. Holes of this kind vary in size from those with a diameter of two or three millimetres to others with a diameter of a centimetre or even more. Depending partly on the size of the hole, blood in amounts ranging from one and a half litres to five litres a minute is shunted directly from the left ventricle where the pressure is high to the right ventricle where it is lower (left to right shunt). As a result the right ventricle becomes overfilled and has to circulate larger amounts of blood through the lungs and back to the left heart. All the affected chambers, the right ventricle, the left atrium and the left ventricle are overloaded and consequently become enlarged. In spite of this a reasonably effective circulation can be maintained for some time, perhaps for years. Eventually the heart muscle weakens and the heart begins to fail (see Chapter 3). Sometimes the increased volume of blood in the pulmonary circulation provokes narrowing of the smaller pulmonary arteries (vaso constriction) increasing the resistance in the pulmonary circulation and causing the pulmonary arterial pressure to rise. It may even reach a level equal to that in the systemic arteries. In such circumstances the shunt may be "reversed" so that blood flows from the right ventricle to the left as well as from the left ventricle to the right with the consequences discussed above – a blue baby.

A hole between the atria (atrial septal defect) is generally large with a diameter of 1 to 3 centimetres. This allows free communication of blood at that level. The greater pressure in the left atrium directs blood through the hole into the right heart so that the right atrium, the right ventricle and the pulmonary arteries become overfilled and enlarged. Because the shunt takes place in the atria the abnormal pressures are not as great as with a ventricular septal defect and the effects on the heart are less severe. Patients with atrial septal defects, although limited in their capacity for physical exertion are likely to experience long periods of good health often reaching middle age before the heart begins to fail.

Malformed pulmonary arteries

Failure to separate the aorta and the pulmonary artery nearly always leads to narrowing (stenosis) of the pulmonary artery which is sometimes too poorly developed to allow blood to flow through it (pulmonary atresia: see explanations). Sometimes the narrowing can occur at the level of the pulmonary valves but more often it involves the whole stem of the artery as it leaves the heart. In this latter case the defect is likely to be combined with other abnormalities such as a defect in the interventricular septum (partition between the ventricles) and an aorta which originates partly from the left and partly from the right ventricle. Inevitably in such cases the pressure becomes the same in both ventricles with the above normal pressure this involves for the right ventricle causing it to enlarge and hypertrophy.

The combination of these four abnormalities was described in 1888 by a French physician Fallot and is known as Fallot's tetralogy (a group of four) or sometimes for short as a "Fallot". It is probably the commonest cause of a blue baby.

Pulmonary stenosis at valve level is generally a less serious condition and may often be an isolated defect which causes little trouble until well into adult life. By then the continued strain on the right ventricle resulting from the abnormal resistance to flow through the narrowed valve may lead to a degree of heart failure. Sometimes in such cases the pressure in the right ventricle is exceptionally high and this may either prevent the closure of the foramen ovale at birth or cause it to open again after it has closed. In both cases there can then be a right to left shunt with cyanosis.

Malformed Aorta

Malformations of the aorta are less common than malformations of the pulmonary artery but two of them are important. Valves with one or two cusps instead of the normal three may be the site of thrombosis in adult life and lead to stenosis (described on page 45). Severe narrowing of the aorta near its origin (coarctation) may prevent the blood reaching the lower part of the body in the normal way. Although alternative channels usually open up to by-pass the obstruction they are less efficient than normal and sometimes fail to supply the kidneys properly with blood. Consequently high blood pressure develops, usually at a fairly early age (see under High Blood Pressure Chapter 5).

Patent ductus arteriosus

Before birth there is a short communicating channel between the aorta and pulmonary artery called the ductus arteriosus. Its function is to ensure that blood which, after birth, would be oxygenated in the lungs is returned to the placenta to receive oxygen. Normally it closes when the lungs begin to function immediately after birth. Sometimes it remains open (patent). Blood is then diverted directly from the aorta to the pulmonary artery. A small patent ductus arteriosus, as it is called medically, may have very little effect on the heart and circulation but generally the shunt occurring in this way is substantial. The pulmonary arteries overfill, more blood is returned to the left heart, which in due course enlarges and eventually begins to fail usually in early adolescence. Sometimes the increased pulmonary blood flow stimulates active constriction of the smaller arteries and raises the pulmonary artery pressure with consequences similar to those occurring in one type of hole in the heart (ventricular septal defect) explained from page 53.

PROSPECTS FOR CONGENITAL ABNORMALITIES AND VALVULAR DISEASE

Left to themselves these abnormalities tend to run the kind of course described in each case. They are often compatible with fair or even normal health for some years and even when they do cause trouble they can still be improved by treatment. Moreover advances in surgery over the past 30 years have offered the prospects of virtual cure in a number of conditions and greatly altered the situation. More is said about them in Chapter 7.

PERICARDIAL DISEASE

Inflammation affecting the underlying heart muscle often spreads to the pericardium – the sac in which the heart is situated – and is known as pericarditis. This is particularly so in Rheumatic Fever or with direct infection by bacteria or viruses. Virus diseases such as Glandular Fever, inflammatory diseases of uncertain origin, and tuberculosis sometimes affect the pericardium itself. Damage (infarction) to the superficial parts of the heart muscle after a coronary thrombosis nearly always affects the adjacent pericardium. Other diseases, including inflammation and tumours may spread from adjoining structures in the chest such as the lungs and pleura.

Disease of the pericardium nearly always causes pain not unlike that of Angina though generally more localised. Fever and a fast pulse are to be expected with acute inflammation but otherwise the heart's action may be unaffected. However a liability of pericardial inflammation (and indeed of inflammation in similar structures such as the pleura covering the lungs and the peritoneum covering the gut) is the outpouring of fluid, sometimes in large amounts, into the pericardial sac. This can lead to a condition in which the heart is prevented by the pressure in the pericardium from expanding and filling properly, known as "cardiac tamponade". Consequently the pressure in the great veins entering the heart rises causing enlargement of the liver, dropsy (see page 67) and accumulation of fluid in the pleural cavities. When the pulmonary veins are also affected there is congestion of the lungs. In severe cases the output of the heart and the blood pressure fall, sometimes dangerously, unless the fluid is promptly removed.

Constrictive Pericarditis

An important although rather rare form of pericarditis is known as constrictive pericarditis. In this condition which is caused by chronic inflammation, particularly by tuberculosis, the heart becomes encased in a mass of chronic inflammatory tissue which is generally calcified (see explanations). The pericardial sac is all but obliterated and the heart is permanently constricted. As a result the pressures in the systemic and pulmonary veins are permanently raised with the consequences just mentioned. Constrictive pericarditis can be relieved only by surgical operation.

Treatment of disease of the heart

Some diseases of the heart do not need treatment; there are others for which no effective treatment exists. Where disease is detected the first rule is to decide whether it is affecting the function of the heart or whether it is likely to do so in the near future. If so the disordered function must be treated on lines which will be described in Chapter 7. Heart muscle damage always needs treatment appropriate to the disease causing it and a period of rest until it has been controlled. Bacterial Endocarditis and suspected Bacterial Endocarditis need urgent treatment with appropriate antibiotics. Coronary Heart Disease needs rest and management, often in hospital in the acute phase, and measures designed to prevent its extension in the future. Valvular Disease, Congenital Abnormalities and Constrictive Pericarditis should always be considered for possible surgical correction. High Blood Pressure must be managed along lines which will be discussed in Chapter 5. Complete heart block (see page 65) with very slow ventricular rates can often be strikingly improved by a permanent artificial pacemaker. Treatment is discussed in greater detail in Chapter 7.

3
WHAT HAPPENS WHEN THE HEART GOES WRONG

Heart disease causes no trouble unless it interferes with the way in which the heart works. There are three ways in which this can happen each of which can cause symptoms. They are *disorders of the heart beat, heart pain* (Angina Pectoris) and *heart failure*. There are also symptoms which are mistakenly attributed to heart trouble.

All of these are discussed in detail in this chapter or later but first let us clear up a popular misconception about heart failure. Laymen usually think that this term means the heart has stopped and that life is at an end. This can be the cause of some misery until they understand how doctors use the term differently. Their meaning is nearly always only that the heart is beginning to show signs of strain and finding difficulty in meeting all the demands on the circulation. This is very different and a long way from the end.

The ways in which heart trouble can be detected and corrected or improved are discussed in Chapters 6 and 7.

Explanation of how an electrocardiogram – a key diagnostic tool – is prepared will be found in detail in Chapter 6. Meanwhile Figs. 6–9 reveal what the E.C.G. will show where flutter or fibrillation are present, compared to normal results.

DISORDERS OF THE HEART BEAT

Disorders of the heart beat often occur in people with healthy hearts. They can be associated with heart disease but even then they are not necessarily serious, although sometimes they can lead to heart failure. Minor disorders are often unnoticed but they may cause discomfort and anxiety. Generally disorders of the heart beat are of two kinds. In one the normal pacemaker's control of the heart is interrupted by occasional beats arising from an abnormal focus of activation. In the other an abnormal focus of activation takes over completely either temporarily or permanently from the normal pacemaker.

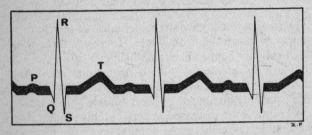

Fig. 6 Normal electrocardiogram showing three consecutive heart beats.

Extra beats

Occasional out of place beats interrupting normal pacemaker control (ectopic beats: extra systoles) can be activated from any part of the heart including the atria, the atrio-ventricular node, and the ventricles. Generally they make the heart beat a fraction of a second before it is due (premature beat). This usually blocks the next normally activated beat. If it comes too quickly after the preceding normal heart beat, ectopic activity either fails to induce a heart beat or else induces one which does not send enough blood from the heart to produce an arterial pulse. The result is a missed beat.

Extra beats are sometimes felt as a jump or a double beat in the chest but often they are not noticed at all. Doctors can usually diagnose them by feeling the pulse and listening to the heart at the same time. Sometimes an electrocardiogram is necessary. How this is done is explained on page 112.

The mechanism responsible for extra beats is complex but the majority occur in people with healthy hearts. Sometimes they seem to be brought on by smoking, by drinking alcohol or by anxiety, and sometimes by disease in neighbouring parts of the body such as the chest or the stomach. They are often found in people taking drugs such as digitalis and they can be a sign of muscle damage, especially if they arise in the ventricle (see Chapter 4).

By themselves extra beats are not harmful. Their significance depends upon their cause.

Intermittent disorders
(Paroxysmal tachycardias: see explanations)

These are disorders of rhythm caused by temporary replacement of the normal pacemaker by a series of discharges from an abnormal focus which may be either short lived or long lasting. Generally the abnormal focus of activation, which may be situated in any part of the heart, discharges regular impulses at a rate between 140 and 200 or higher. (This compares with a normal rate of 70 heart beats per minute in someone sitting quietly.) As a rule the heart responds by beating regularly at the high rate.

Characteristically these disorders start abruptly and often without any obvious precipitating cause. They may last either for a few beats or for long periods varying from a

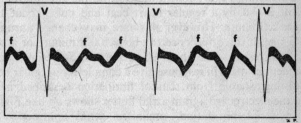

Fig. 7 Electrocardiogram: Atrial flutter showing fast regular atrial activity (f) and slower ventricular response (V).

few hours to days or rarely weeks. Often they appear to stop gradually. This is because the heart beat remains rather fast for a time after normal pacemaker control has been restored. Provided that the heart is otherwise healthy and provided that the attacks do not last too long paroxysmal tachycardias are generally well tolerated. The rapid heart beat is usually felt immediately and may be uncomfortable. It is generally described as palpitation. Attacks may be associated with breathlessness on exertion and sometimes with faintness especially when they first come on. Experienced sufferers, however, can sometimes continue physical activities such as playing cricket. Paroxysmal tachycardias can be a sign of other heart disease, especially when they arise from a focus in the ventricles but the majority occur without demonstrable cause. They may recur repeatedly but are generally compatible with good health and a normal life span.

Other disorders

Two other heart beat disorders in which normal pacemaker control is displaced are atrial flutter and atrial fibrillation. In flutter the heart is believed to be activated by an atrial focus which discharges very rapid and regular impulses at a rate between 250 and 350 times a minute. Although the ventricles sometimes respond to each impulse they are more likely to respond to every second or third and sometimes every fourth impulse. At the initial level the result is usually a regular heart beat and pulse about 150 times a minute. However this rate may change abruptly to a one in three response of about 100 a minute or a one in four response at about 75 a minute. Sometimes very frequent changes in response give a completely irregular beat indistinguishable from that of fibrillation described next. On the electrocardiagram atrial flutter shows up like Fig. 7.

In atrial fibrillation, organised atrial contraction is replaced by patchy, irregular and extremely rapid activation of the muscle with the result that a normal effective atrial

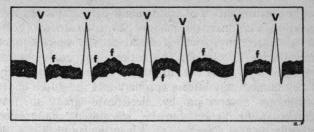

Fig. 8 Electrocardiogram: Atrial fibrillation; poorly defined irregular atrial activity (f), fast irregular ventricular response (V).

contraction rarely takes place. Because ventricular filling is impaired and ventricular contraction erratic, the heart beat is fast and unpredictable with an output which varies from beat to beat. Look at Fig. 8.

Both atrial flutter and atrial fibrillation can occur in paroxysms but sooner or later they tend to become permanent. Flutter seldom stays unchanged for long even when established, and tends to alter spontaneously to fibrillation. Both disorders are likely to be associated with heart muscle disease.

Atrial flutter and persistent atrial fibrillation tend to cause some degree of heart failure unless they are controlled by treatment. A potentially serious complication sometimes associated with fibrillation is the formation of blood clots in the heart because of pooling of blood in the poorly contracting atria. These can be discharged into the circulation where they can block arteries in distant parts of the body (embolism) with characteristic effects (see Chapter 2). Atrial fibrillation is often found in old people who are apparently well; the heart beat is usually slower and the condition causes little trouble.

Ventricular fibrillation

This grave disorder occurs usually as a terminal event in long-standing disease of the ventricular muscle although it can be a complication of acute muscle damage such as that caused by a coronary thrombosis. Normal ventricular beating is replaced by patchy irregular activity which cannot maintain the circulation. The patient loses consciousness and there is no heart beat or pulse. People are particularly at risk immediately after a coronary and should be under continuous observation by electrocardiogram so that ventricular fibrillation can be recognised and treated immediately (see Chapter 6). A ventricular fibrillation is shown by the electrocardiogram in Fig. 9.

Disorders of conduction (heart block)

Disorders can occur at any level in the conducting system. Either the atrio-ventricular bundle as referred to in Chapter 1 or one of its branches are most likely to be affected. This delays or sometimes interrupts the spread of the excitation process in the heart and is called heart block. Delay or occasional interruption of the spread of the excitation process from the atrium to the ventricle is known as "partial heart block". Delay or interruption in one of the branches of the conducting system is also known as "bundle branch block". Partial heart block may cause the ventricle to miss

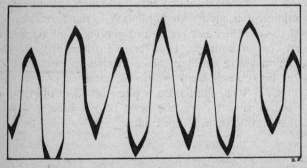

Fig. 9. Electrocardiogram: Ventricular fibrillation. Disorganised ventricular activity (deflections shown better formed and slower than usual).

a beat with a corresponding missed arterial pulse but it is unlikely to interfere with the function of the heart. Bundle branch block causes delayed activation of the ventricle on the affected side and this interferes with the normal nearly synchronous contraction of the ventricles. By itself it has little effect on heart function but it can be an indication of muscle disease. Partial heart block and Bundle Branch block are both generally detected by an electrocardiogram.

In "complete heart block" the ventricles are cut off from normal pacemaker control. When this happens they beat with a slow regular rate usually between 30 and 40 times a minute but sometimes much more slowly. This can cause trouble. For one thing the long interval between beats predisposes to overfilling of the heart and imposes an additional load which may lead to enlargement and eventually to some heart failure. More likely are attacks of fairly sudden loss of consciousness caused by failure of the circulation to the brain, either because of cessation (standstill) of the heart beat or because of the onset of an abnormal ventricular rhythm or because of both in combination. Attacks of this kind (Stokes Adams attacks) are usually brief and generally recover completely, but they tend to recur without warning and are sometimes fatal. Their treatment by artificial pacemakers is discussed in Chapter 7.

HEART PAIN

Unless the pericardium is involved heart disease is seldom associated with pain. The important exception is the pain of Angina Pectoris and of coronary thrombosis which is nearly always the result of disease of the coronary arteries causing interference with the blood supply to the heart. It will be discussed in the next chapter more fully.

HEART FAILURE

The most serious form of heart trouble is heart failure but as emphasised to begin this chapter it is important to understand what this means. It does not normally when talked of by a doctor mean that the heart has stopped and that life has come to an end. Sometimes this does happen but usually what the doctor means is that the capacity of the heart to meet all demands on the circulation has become limited because of disease. This certainly imposes restrictions and possibly frustration but it is a long way from the end of life.

In terms of the circulation, heart failure means that the heart is generally managing to maintain a normal or nearly normal output of blood at rest but is unable to meet extra demands. It may not supply enough blood to the kidneys with consequent increase in blood volume and distention and enlargement of the heart and great veins. The pressure in the veins entering the failing chamber or chambers rises and is responsible for the clinical effects which will be explained as you read on. Extra physical exertion makes heart failure worse, as do other bodily diseases such as infection, especially in the lungs, and anaemia. These must be treated appropriately if they are present.

Heart failure itself can nearly always be improved and sometimes greatly improved by treatment even though this may not, and generally does not, cure the underlying disease. Eventually of course unless the underlying disease can be cured, working under handicap in this way imposes further strains on the heart. Finally it does stop. This may not happen for a long time and before it does a reasonably satisfying and even nearly normal life can often be enjoyed.

The pattern of heart failure varies according to the side of the heart which is predominantly affected. Though both sides are usually affected in the long run it is convenient to describe their effects separately.

Right heart failure

A failing right heart causes the pressure to rise in the great veins bringing blood back from the body (the central venous pressure). This is transmitted through all the systemic veins and notably to those draining the liver and the kidneys. In people with a failing right heart the neck veins (the jugular veins) become distended and can be seen pulsating at a higher level than normal, and the liver becomes enlarged and sometimes painful. Effects on the kidneys cause retention of salt and water in the body which further overloads the circulation. In due course fluid escapes from the circulation and accumulates in the soft tissues causing dropsy (oedema). Under the influence of gravity the lower limbs in people who are up and about and the lower part of the back in people in bed become swollen. Although popularly regarded as the outstanding sign of a failing heart dropsy is generally preceded by other symptoms and occurs at a rather advanced stage.

Right sided heart failure is often the result of gradual failure of the left heart since the raised pressures which this produces in the pulmonary circulation are liable to affect the right heart. It may be also caused by lung diseases such as bronchitis and emphysema (see explanations). Less often disease of its own valves (the pulmonary and tricuspid valves) may be responsible.

A severe and acute (sudden) form of right heart failure may follow obstruction of a pulmonary artery or one of its branches. It is usually caused by a thrombus or part of a thrombus which has formed in a deep vein, perhaps in the leg, and has been swept into the right heart and thence into a pulmonary artery or one of its branches (pulmonary embolism, see explanations). It is a complication of prolonged bed rest for illnesses such as a coronary thrombosis, and of some surgical operations. Pulmonary artery obstruction of this kind raises the pressure in the pulmonary artery sharply and suddenly. The right heart is unable to overcome this and cannot therefore supply a proper amount of blood to the left heart. In consequence the output of the left heart fails rapidly, the pulse volume diminishes, the blood pressure falls and the person affected becomes pale, cold and drowsy. The condition may be fatal unless quickly relieved.

Left heart failure

A failing left heart causes a rise of pressure in the pulmonary veins. Eventually fluid escapes into the lungs which become progressively stiffer and in very severe cases nearly waterlogged. As a result people affected become breathless, at first during exercise, and later if the disorder is allowed to progress, when sitting still and particularly when lying down.

When the left heart fails gradually as it usually does both the left atrium and the left ventricle are involved. This tends to raise the pressure gradually in the pulmonary circulation and in due course to cause right as well as left heart failure.

"Cardiac Asthma". (Left ventricular failure)

When disease of the left heart is confined to the left ventricle as with aortic valve obstruction, and sometimes with high blood pressure and where failure is fairly rapid, the pulmonary circulation becomes acutely congested with blood. This causes a particularly severe condition known as "Cardiac Asthma". Coming on characteristically during sleep, cardiac asthma wakes the patient in a state of severe breathlessness not unlike a severe asthmatic attack. He may rush to a window for air. Generally the attack passes off after periods of time lasting up to an hour. Sometimes minor warning attacks precede a full blown attack and may be mistaken for bad dreams. Even a full blown attack may be repeated once or twice before it is recognised for what it is and treated.

Normally when people lie down more blood comes into the right heart, the filling pressure rises and more blood is pumped through the lungs into the left heart. The healthy left ventricle deals with this without difficulty but is unable to do so when weakened by disease. As long as the right heart remains healthy it continues to pump blood through the lungs and the pressure in the pulmonary veins rises sharply. Fluid escapes rapidly into the lungs causing severe shortness of breath. A person lying down and awake would automatically want to sit up if he felt breathless and would thus reduce the filling pressure in the heart and relieve the congestion of the lungs. In sleep the congestion builds up unnoticed until it has become severe. In acute left sided failure of this kind, right sided heart failure, though not present at first, generally comes on sooner or later and the patient then becomes more comfortable because the output of the two ventricles is then balanced, albeit at a lower level.

Left heart failure is usually caused by longstanding disease either of the mitral or aortic valves or by sustained high blood pressure. Sudden and severe damage to the left ventricle immediately after a coronary thrombosis (see Chapter 4) sometimes causes a different condition from that just described. It is known as shock.

Shock

Spoken of by doctors as "cardiogenic shock" to distinguish it from the term popularly used in states of fear or sudden emotional upset and from the description of other kinds of circulatory collapse such as those caused by severe loss of blood, or through severe generalised infections, shock is caused by a sudden and severe fall in the output of blood from the left ventricle. The blood pressure falls and the supply of blood to all parts of the body is reduced. Compensatory measures come into play and divert blood from the skin and the muscles in order to protect vital organs such as the brain, the kidneys and the heart itself. As with pulmonary embolism the person feels faint, becomes pale and cold, and may lose consciousness. Particularly severe shock may cause sudden death because of failure of the circulation to the brain. The condition is always serious and a low output may persist for some days. The heart may stop suddenly. Treatment is discussed in Chapter 7. The long term outlook depends upon the severity of the muscle damage causing the reduced output from the left ventricle.

SYMPTOMS MISTAKEN FOR HEART TROUBLE

Fainting attacks

A faint is a loss of consciousness caused by temporary failure of the blood supply to the brain. There are a number of ways in which fainting can occur and the character of the attack may differ slightly with each of them. The majority of fainting attacks are *not* caused by heart disease, although heart conditions such as sudden severe heart failure (shock), complete heart block, disorders of the heart beat and obstructive disease of the aortic valve are all liable to be associated with fainting.

Other symptoms

Other symptoms mistaken for heart trouble are pain in the left side of the chest, and palpitation.

Left sided chest pain is quite unlike true heart pain (angina). It is often felt as a dull ache, with or without occasional momentary stabs of pain in the place where the heart is thought to be. Unlike Angina it is as a rule unrelated to exertion and may last continuously for hours at a time. Angina never does that without having serious effects on the circulation. Furthermore angina occurs in the centre of the chest and is a hard, pressing or tight sensation nearly always coming on during exercise and stopping fairly quickly afterwards. Left chest pain has a number of causes of which myalgia (see explanations) or neuralgia of the chest wall, possibly aggravated by fear of heart disease, are the most likely.

Palpitation is an undue awareness of the heart beat either because it is quicker or more forcible than normal. There are many causes. The rapid heart beat occurring when you run upstairs or run for a bus sometimes causes palpitation which goes on for a time after you have stopped running. It is particularly noticeable if you are not fit. Mental tension and anxiety sometimes make the heart beat more forcibly for a time. Often it is worse lying down at night when the beat can sometimes be heard. Palpitation is not usually a sign of heart trouble unless it is caused by a disorder of the heart beat such as paroxysmal tachycardia or atrial fibrillation. Then it is very fast and sometimes irregular.

Another symptom causing unnecessary alarm may falsely be described as *breathlessness*. In fact it is more a sensation of being unable to take a full breath, or a sighing sensation. It is generally unlike the breathlessness when someone with early heart failure over-exerts himself.

A well known condition originally mistaken for heart trouble occurred during the First World War and was known as "Soldier's Heart" because it affected young soldiers when undergoing military training. Its main features were a rather rapid and forcible heart beat of over 100 per minute accompanied by a constant dull ache in the left chest. Sufferers tired easily and complained of being breathless during the kind of exercise that normal people could undertake without serious difficulty. Similar symptoms were reported in the Second World War when they were generally called "Effort Syndrome". Most of the people affected had been living rather sheltered lives in peace time because they were incapable of doing anything else. Some of them became normal after a period of graduated physical training. Others continued to have symptoms which were sometimes disabling. People with symptoms of this kind seem to have a constitutional weakness of the circulatory system just as other people seem to have a constitutionally weak stomach – but they are not suffering from heart disease. Quite often they have been brought up in families centering round a father's or mother's heart disease and may have gone about in fear of heart disease all their lives. Fortunately symptoms are seldom as bad as those occurring during the War. More often they come and go, sometimes shortly after periods of stress or depression. They can usually be relieved by firm and decisive reassurance. Psychiatric treatment is rarely necessary unless such people are severely depressed.

4
CORONARY
HEART DISEASE

SUMMARY

Coronary heart disease is the result of damage to the coronary arteries which reduces their capacity to supply the heart with blood. The damage is caused by a complex disease process. No single cause has been found but a number of predisposing associations have been established. They include a high level of fat in the blood, possibly caused by eating too much of the wrong kind of food, heavy cigarette smoking, a Westernised life style, and a familial liability. The detailed findings are to be found later in this chapter.

Coronary heart disease shows itself either as Angina Pectoris or as a "coronary" (coronary thrombosis). Angina is a specific pain in the chest occurring generally during exercise. A coronary is a sudden and sometimes severe illness caused by acute damage to the heart muscle. We concentrate next on their specific recognition and management.

Coronary heart disease is the commonest and most important form of heart muscle disease. Together with High Blood Pressure which often goes with it, it causes the greatest number of deaths in advanced or affluent and industrialised societies. It is also responsible for much serious ill health and anxiety.

In Great Britain alone disease of the heart and arteries is responsible for almost half the deaths in men and women between 45 and 55 and about three quarters of them are caused by coronary heart disease. The proportion in men between 35 and 45 is rather smaller but is still appreciable. Its incidence was greatly reduced during the War but the last twenty years have seen a steady increase affecting younger people particularly. Pathological examinations after death have suggested that as many as thirty per cent of middle aged men in Britain have evidence of coronary artery disease.

CAUSES OF CORONARY HEART DISEASE

Numerous attempts have been made and continue to be made to isolate the factors responsible. Diet, cigarette smoking, and lack of exercise have all attracted their share of blame and so have the reactions of certain personality types to the general way of life and "stress" of Westernised societies. However coronary heart disease stems from coronary artery disease, and circumstantial evidence however valid statistically, cannot be entirely acceptable unless it can be directly related to the disease processes involved. These are atheroma and thrombosis. Although different in nature they are undoubtedly closely related and some authorities believe that atheroma is directly caused by thrombosis. Atheroma (Greek: porridge) is a descriptive term denoting the presence of fatty material in the arterial wall. This hardens and distorts the artery and narrows its channel. Thrombosis in this context means the formation of a thrombus (see later heading in this chapter) in the arterial channel.

Atheroma, sometimes loosely spoken of as "arteriosclerosis", is patchily distributed throughout the coronary arteries but particularly affects the left coronary artery and its descending branch which supply the greater part of the left ventricle. It is generally believed to be caused by infiltration of the arterial wall by fats which are circulating in the blood. This provokes a cellular reaction which affects the artery in the way just stated. How and why it happens is not entirely clear but the process seems to be gradual, probably lasting over a period of years and perhaps even starting in childhood.

The blood fats

The blood fats consist of four main substances. They are *fatty acids, neutral fats (triglycerides)* consisting of three molecules of a fatty acid combined with glycerol, *phospholipids* containing fatty acids, phosphorous and a nitrogenous base, and *cholesterol*.

Fatty acids are substances in which chains of carbon atoms of varying length are linked to hydrogen atoms and to oxygen. They are either "saturated" or "unsaturated". Unsaturated fatty acids may have one double linkage (mono-unsaturated) or more than one double linkage (poly-unsaturated) between carbon atoms, and this enables them to bind additional hydrogen and other atoms. Saturated fatty acids have no such double linkage. Of the blood fats palmitic and stearic acids are saturated and oleic acid is unsaturated. Certain poly-unsaturated fatty acids such as arachidonic acid, linoleic acid, and linolenic acid are necessary to bodily growth and development and are therefore known as essential fatty acids. Arachidonic acid can be made in the body from linoleic acid, but linoleic and linolenic acid cannot and must be supplied in the diet. Cholesterol is based on carbon atoms arranged in rings and circulates either as free cholesterol or in combination with a fatty acid (cholesterol ester).

Fat transport in the blood

With the exception of phospholipids fats are insoluble in the blood and have to be transported in combination with protein. These combined fats are known as lipoproteins. They vary considerably in molecular weight and in density. One way of separating them according to their density is to centrifuge them at high speed (ultracentrifugation) in a salt solution with a specific gravity above that of water (1.063). After centrifugation low density lipoproteins tend to float and high density lipoproteins tend to sink. Low density lipoproteins contain relatively large amounts of fat and cholesterol. High density lipoproteins contain relatively little.

The distribution of lipoproteins in the blood varies in different populations and is probably genetically determined. It is also affected by age, sex, body weight and diet, and perhaps by the amount of exercise taken. In general, men below the age of fifty have lower levels of high density lipoproteins than women. After the age of fifty the differences tend to disappear and the pattern in men becomes more like that in women. A diet sufficient to maintain a steady body weight with the calories derived from 15% protein, 45% fat and 45% carbohydrates will generally maintain a "normal" lipoprotein distribution. Excessive dietary calories and diets containing large amounts of saturated fat or large amounts of carbohydrate increase the proportion of lower density lipoprotein. Substituting poly-unsaturated fats for saturated fats in the diet generally reduces the lower density lipoproteins. Regular exercise and a moderate intake of some forms of alcohol, such as wine, have been thought to increase the high density lipoproteins. Heavy smoking and possibly heavy consumption of alcohol tend to increase the proportion of low density lipoproteins.

The way in which fats are transported may play an important part in the production of coronary artery disease. Fat transported in low density lipoproteins seems to be readily deposited in the arterial wall. High density lipoproteins on the other hand seem to clear fats from the arterial wall.

Source and bodily use of blood fats

Blood fats are derived partly from food and are partly made in the body. Fatty acids, mostly saturated, are contained in meat, dairy products, especially butter, and in cooking fats (visible fats) but also in substances such as chocolate, some cheeses and potato crisps (non-visible fats).

Unsaturated fatty acids are found in certain vegetable oils, such as corn oil, sunflower and safflower oil, and in some fish oils such as mackerel oil and whale oil much consumed by Eskimos. They are also contained in some soft margarine. Cholesterol is present in meat, dairy products, particularly in butter and cream, in egg yolk and in chocolate.

Food fats appear in the blood after digestion mainly as triglycerides and in lesser amounts as free fatty acids; that is as acids unattached to any other substance. Fatty acids are a major source of body energy. They have a short life in the blood and are either broken down to provide energy or converted into triglycerides and stored in the fat deposits of the body (adipose tissue). Carbohydrate is also converted to fat and similarly stored. Storage is not a static process because triglycerides are being constantly mobilised and broken down into free fatty acids and glycerol to supply energy. Utilisation of fat in this way depends largely upon a readily available supply of carbohydrates. Adrenaline and noradrenaline secreted by sympathetic nerves and by the supra-renal glands play an important part in the breakdown of triglycerides into free fatty acids.

The normal function of cholesterol is not well understood. It is one of the main building blocks of the body, particularly important in cell walls; it is also a constituent of many tissues notably of the supra-renal glands and of the sex hormones. An average European diet contains about 600 milligrams of cholesterol a day and provides about one fifth of the circulating cholesterol. The remainder is made in the body mainly in the liver. The synthesis of this "endogenous" cholesterol is regulated partly by the amount of cholesterol in the blood derived from the diet and partly by the availability of sugar and insulin. Cholesterol as well as being made in the liver is broken down there when required and converted chiefly into bile acids. See also next section.

Thrombosis

Thrombosis may occur in almost any part of the cardio-vascular system. It is commonest in veins and in arteries but it can also occur on the heart valves and on the inner walls of the heart chambers, especially when the muscle is damaged.

Thrombus formation (thrombosis) sometimes popularly thought of as clot formation is in fact complex and depends essentially upon a cellular element of the blood, the blood platelets. Under certain circumstances these can adhere to the inner wall for example of an artery, particularly where it is damaged. They can also aggregate in clumps. Aggregation (clumping) depends upon a balance of chemical factors in the blood some of which promote and some of which inhibit it. Important substances tending to promote aggregation are adrenaline and noradrenaline. Another is thromboxane which is formed in platelets and is released into the blood when they aggregate. A further derivative of the essential poly-unsaturated fatty acid arachidonic acid is known as prostacyclin. This is formed in blood vessel walls and tends to inhibit platelet aggregation. Diets containing large amounts of poly-unsaturated fats therefore tend to have a similar inhibitory effect. Drugs such as aspirin tend to inhibit aggregation probably by interfering with the release of thromboxane. On the other hand a high level of blood fat, especially of cholesterol, promotes both platelet aggregation and platelet adhesion. A single fatty meal temporarily inhibits the formation of factors opposing platelet aggregation.

Thrombosis in an artery occurs rapidly, probably within hours or at the most days. It is particularly likely to occur where an artery gives off one of its branches or where its wall has been damaged by pre-existing disease. Thrombosis in an artery begins when platelets adhere to the inner wall of the vessel. Clumping takes place and attracts other platelets to the site. Secondary blood clotting follows and a protein (fibrin) and other cellular elements of the blood become trapped in a growing cellular mass which if it is large enough can obstruct the arterial channel or even block it completely (this is the usual cause of a "coronary"). In due course the thrombus shrinks and becomes incorporated into the arterial wall but it generally leaves permanent damage which distorts the vessel.

Food fats, blood fats and coronary heart disease

The belief that the main cause of coronary heart disease is atheroma, and that atheroma depends directly on the amount of fat, particularly cholesterol, circulating in the blood is strongly held by many authorities. The amount of fat in the blood is believed to depend on the amount of fat, particularly of saturated fat in the diet. Large scale studies seem to support this. They have shown that populations with a high prevalence of coronary heart disease have high levels of circulating cholesterol and to a lesser extent of triglycerides and tend to consume diets rich in saturated fats. No critical level of cholesterol has been determined and the liability is relative. The higher the blood fats, particularly cholesterol, the more coronary heart disease; the lower the blood fats the less coronary heart disease. The findings apply particularly to men below 60 years of age. Similar findings have emerged from studies of groups within populations.

That the high blood cholesterol is the result of diet and of social habits and is not genetic in origin is supported by the finding that groups of people migrating from countries where cholesterol levels are low and where the prevalence of coronary heart disease is low to those where both are high acquire the characteristics of their new environment – namely high blood cholesterol and a high prevalence of coronary heart disease.

In spite of impressive evidence of this kind cholesterol and dietary habits do not seem to be reliable predictors of individual liability to disease. People with diseases such as diabetes, where the blood cholesterol and the blood fats are often high, and where fat metabolism is often disturbed are certainly prone to coronary heart disease. The same is true, though perhaps to a lesser degree with thyroid deficiency (Myxoedema) and with a form of kidney disease (nephrosis) in both of which the blood cholesterol is high. Also a rather rare familial disorder where the blood cholesterol is exceptionally high carries a greatly increased risk not only of coronary heart disease but of generalised arterial disease. However diseases of this kind account for only a small proportion of coronary heart disease. A more recent version of the rôle of blood fats may be nearer the mark. Because fat transported in high density lipoproteins is less likely to be deposited in the arterial wall than fat transported in low density lipoproteins it suggests that the ratio of high density lipoproteins to total cholesterol in the blood may be a better predictor of liability to coronary heart disease than the absolute levels of cholesterol.

Objections to the emphasis on the rôle of food fats

For a number of reasons some authorities are sceptical about the rôle of blood and food fats. As stated above cholesterol levels are not reliable predictors of individual liability to coronary heart disease. Furthermore the relationship between cholesterol levels and the incidence of heart disease is complex and needs to be adjusted for age. At best it seems to show that those with high and very high levels are at risk. Individuals react surprisingly differently to fat in the diet. A diet rich in saturated fat or in cholesterol will produce strikingly high levels of blood cholesterol in some people but will be virtually without effect in others. Food is in any case responsible for only about one fifth of the blood cholesterol. The remainder is made in the body and depends on other factors including the consumption of refined carbohydrate such as sugar. In this connection it is interesting to note that dietary fibre, mostly in the form of wheat fibre (bran) and long advocated as "roughage" for the prevention of constipation and other intestinal disorders is believed by some to protect against coronary heart disease. If this is true it could be because it can slow the absorption of fat from food but equally it could be the result of its ability to delay the absorption of sugar and so to reduce the amount of cholesterol made in the body. Insistence upon the value of unsaturated fats in lowering the blood cholesterol has also been criticised because at least one of these is known to raise it and because the only unsaturated fats known to lower it consistently are the essential fatty acids, arachidonic, linoleic and linolenic acids. In practice however extensive trials in the U.S.A., Sweden and Finland have shown that the blood cholesterol can be lowered by 10% to 15% by diets rich in poly-unsaturated fats and by drugs. Doing this appears to have reduced the incidence of non-fatal coronary heart disease in apparently healthy people including those with high or very high levels of blood cholesterol. The effect of the diets on fatal coronary disease is less certain.

The role of fats in the blood and the food might indeed be better understood if more attention was paid to their effects on thrombosis and if they were studied more closely in relation to the various forms which coronary heart disease can take.

The whole nutritional concept can be seriously criticised for paying too little attention to thrombosis as a cause of coronary heart disease. Important evidence to support this comes from studies of the Eskimo community who derive their fats from fish oil containing eicosapentaenoic acid which is a derivative of linoleic acid. They are remarkably free from coronary artery disease, have a low blood cholesterol but also reduced platelet aggregation with a tendency to bleed easily. Feeding mackerel daily to European volunteers has produced similar changes in the blood which have been convincingly associated with high levels of eicosapentaenoic acid in the blood and in the platelet walls.

A recent finding of an increased tendency of the blood to clot in people particularly liable to coronary heart disease is another pointer to the part played by thrombosis.

OTHER CONTRIBUTORY FACTORS

Preoccupation with blood fats and with diet should not divert attention from other factors associated with coronary heart disease. A tendency for it to run in families and a tendency to attack heavy cigarette smokers are so strongly associated that they appear to constitute independent risk factors in their own right. In addition high blood pressure, the use of oral contraceptives (see below), obesity, softness of the water supply and excessive consumption of coffee have all been implicated but are probably only partly contributory.

A family tendency generally causes disease relatively early in life, in the 40s and 50s and sometimes earlier. The basic reason is by no means clear. Metabolic abnormalities causing a raised blood cholesterol and less often raised triglycerides are sometimes present and have been found particularly in Finland. High blood pressure (hypertension) is found more often. Usually however there is no obvious explanation and observers have been tempted to look for a common factor in similarity of personalities and of life style.

Cigarette smoking is a firmly established risk factor. Heavy smokers (those consuming more than twenty cigarettes a day) have been said to be twice as likely as non-smokers to suffer from coronary heart disease in their 50s. They also seem more liable to sudden death than other sufferers from coronary heart disease. The causes of the association between cigarette smoking and coronary heart disease and in particular with sudden death in coronary sufferers are not entirely clear. Inhalation of nicotine is known to provoke an immediate but short lasting secretion of adrenaline. This increases the heart rate, and the work of the heart, and also mobilises fatty acids. People habitually smoking more than 15 cigarettes a day have been shown in the long term to have higher circulating levels of cholesterol and of low density lipoproteins and a greater tendency of the blood to clot, than non-smokers. Nicotine interferes with the proper oxygenation of the blood too and so may deprive the heart of oxygen at critical times. Whatever the mechanics concerned there is little doubt that a family predisposition and indulgence in heavy smoking are, each individually, major contributors to coronary heart disease.

High blood pressure is fairly often associated with coronary heart disease. Some observers regard the relationship as fortuitous but it is generally believed that high blood pressure in addition to imposing its own specific strain on the heart and arteries (see Chapter 5) contributes directly to disease of the coronary arteries, possibly by making them more susceptible to fatty infiltration.

Obesity and a sedentary way of life are also associated statistically with an increased mortality from coronary heart disease but are almost certainly not primary contributors. Those who have become fat by over-eating have often thereby also acquired abnormalities such as an excess of blood fats or of low density lipoproteins, in addition perhaps to being habitual heavy cigarette smokers but those who have been fat for most of their lives can be perfectly healthy.

The value of exercise is controversial. A classical study of London bus crews found that drivers were significantly more likely than conductors to develop coronary heart disease. There were no other discriminating factors and it seemed proper to conclude that the conductors were protected by the exercise involved in their job. On the other hand studies of athletes have given equivocal results. Marathon runners and others who take regular and prolonged exercise seem relatively free from disease, but the protective value of vigorous sport as a whole is still debated. Exercise has certainly been shown to increase the proportion of high density lipoproteins in the blood in some people but the relative freedom of athletes from other contributory factors such as over-eating and over-smoking may be equally important. However a recent survey of sedentary workers seems to confirm the value of vigorous exercise by itself. Among those studied those who habitually took vigorous spare time exercise either in the form of sport or heavy manual labour had an incidence of coronary heart attacks, and in particular of fatal attacks, over a period of years equal to about half that in those who took no such exercise. The benefit of exercise was especially noticeable in the older members of the group aged between 55 and 65. It was also noticeable even in those who were obese, cigarette smokers, or sufferers from high blood pressure.

Oral contraceptives containing relatively high quantities of ovarian hormones (oestrogens) have been shown to increase the circulating fats and the proportion of low density lipoproteins to total cholesterol and might seem on theoretical grounds to contribute to coronary heart disease. The evidence is indirect but the occurrence of occasional arterial as well as more commonly of venous thrombosis in women taking oral contraceptives is sufficient to raise at least a suspicion that some forms of the pill can contribute to coronary heart disease. They can certainly cause hypertension which usually disappears when they are stopped. There is also clear evidence that pills with a low oestrogen content are less likely to cause venous thrombosis but their effect on the liability to arterial thrombosis is less certain. In practice women over the age of 40 and women of all ages with a family tendency should use oral contraceptives cautiously, especially if they are hypertensive and or heavy cigarette smokers.

Alcohol. The rôle of alcohol in the production of coronary heart disease is debateable. Heavy indulgence does seem to increase the blood fats and low density lipoproteins, possibly by increasing dietary absorption, and to be associated with a higher incidence of coronary heart disease. Moderate drinking on the other hand may be protective partly because it increases the circulating high density lipoproteins and partly because it may stimulate the production of an anti-platelet aggregating substance related to unsaturated fats.

Life style and personality

The belief that certain kinds of people are particularly prone to coronary heart disease is widespread. Tense and aggressive, generally in a hurry and often overweight their eventual "coronary" is accepted by friends and acquaintances as inevitable. More precise analysis of the personality and behaviour of groups of coronary sufferers has given some support to this popular picture. A much publicised study in America identified two types of behaviour in a group of professional men. "Type A" behaviour was characterised by an unusual degree of mental and sometimes physical activity and an intense emotional drive to success often with poorly defined and not easily attainable objectives. Such people also had keenly developed competitive instincts and a desire for recognition and admiration. They were usually working against the clock in an effort to meet impossible deadlines. In contrast "Type B" reactors showed none of these characteristics and lacked the sense of urgency which seemed to go with them. Those with "Type A" behaviour were prone to angina pectoris and to other manifestations of coronary heart disease to which "Type B" people were relatively immune. The initial findings were independent of other contributory factors such as dietary excess and lack of exercise. However subsequent studies have shown that "Type A" people are liable to smoke heavily and to have high levels of blood cholesterol.

The pursuit of material success in industrialised societies demands a high pressure performance which many cannot sustain. "Type A" and similar personalities become easily frustrated when they fail to achieve their aims or when confronted by emotional or financial crises. In such situations, which others accept philosophically or with resignation, they spur themselves to increasing efforts and in the process become tired and steadily less competent. When eventually persuaded, usually by a relative or by business associates, to see a physician they are often on the verge of breakdown. Experienced physicians have detected signs of impending heart strain in such people sufficiently often to believe that unless they change their way of life they are only too likely to suffer a coronary. In spite of criticism on the grounds that this kind of behaviour has been identified only in those of a limited social class and that the characteristics defined could be applied equally to those with high blood pressure or a duodenal ulcer the facts are difficult to ignore.

People with aggressive personalities certainly have a high output of adrenaline and noradrenaline at times of stress. The aggression which sometimes accompanies driving a car or more strikingly racing a car, for example can sometimes provoke a rise in blood pressure and changes in the electrocardiogram. This suggests that temporary impairment of the coronary circulation may be brought about in this way. Longer term studies have shown that people working against the clock secrete and break down more adrenaline and noradrenaline than when doing identical work more or less in their own time.

Adrenaline and noradrenaline play an important part in preparing the body for sudden activity. They are secreted abundantly in times of emergency and in anticipation before a race or some other competitive activity. One of their actions is to break down triglycerides and so to mobilise fatty acids to provide readily available energy. Normally these are consumed in the ensuing physical activity but where they are in excess of bodily requirements they may pave the way for atheroma (explained on page 73). Both adrenaline and noradrenaline also stimulate platelet aggregation and so directly encourage thrombosis. Nevertheless however often acute events of this kind are repeated it is still to be proved that in the long term they can lead to coronary heart disease.

Personal characteristics are notoriously difficult to evaluate but open or overtly aggressive behaviour is not the only psychological association with coronary heart disease. Quiet, tense personalities, perhaps with feelings of frustration and of suppressed hostility also seem liable to be affected, whilst emotional disturbances such as grief have been frequently reported in the weeks immediately preceding a coronary.

A coronary is unfortunately fairly common in previously healthy people shortly after retirement. Possibly the sudden break in an established way of life without any satisfying alternative prospect may in some way precipitate trouble. Overall, however, many coronary patients seem psychologically normal and do not appear to have suffered any particular emotional upset.

SO MANY FACTORS MAY COUNT

Coronary heart disease is the outcome of atheroma and of thrombosis. Both are essentially complex in nature and both are of multifactorial origin. Factors which have been established as contributory to coronary heart disease often influence both processes. Diets for example containing large amounts of saturated fats may increase the amount of fat circulating in the blood and also the low density lipoproteins, both of which are believed to predispose towards infiltration of fat into the arterial wall. At the same time they encourage platelet aggregation and so predispose to thrombosis. Adrenaline and noradrenaline, secreted particularly in times of stress, similarly also influence both processes by mobilising fatty acids from triglycerides and by promoting aggregation of platelets. In contrast a diet containing a high proportion of unsaturated fats, particularly of essential fatty acids, may lower the blood cholesterol. It is also likely to diminish platelet aggregation. Atheroma and thrombosis are so interrelated that they cannot be completely separated. The greater attention now being paid to the factors influencing thrombosis is timely and may help to explain some of the inconsistencies of the nutritional hypothesis.

In practice, extremes of dietary excess (whether of total calories or of saturated fats), heavy cigarette smoking, and persistent aggression (whether overt or suppressed), may all by themselves be capable of causing coronary heart disease, particularly in young men with a family predisposition. The majority of people, however, probably acquire the disease by a combination of more than one contributory factor.

Quite a number of coronary patients indeed appear to show none of the generally accepted characteristics whilst even those showing the greatest number of risk factors only account for about a quarter of those affected. High blood cholesterol levels and heavy cigarette smoking, are undoubtedly independent and valid predictors of disease in large groups of people, but they seem to cause relatively little harm to some individuals and at present we do not know why.

CORONARY HEART DISEASE: SYMPTOMS AND TREATMENT

Heart disease attributable to coronary artery disease shows itself in practice either as Angina Pectoris or as a "coronary".

Angina Pectoris

Angina is a signal that the heart has outrun the supply of oxygen available to it at that moment. As a result chemical products accumulate and stimulate pain producing nerves in the heart muscle. The process continues unless and until the work of the heart is reduced so that the blood supply once more becomes adequate. Angina generally occurs because damaged coronary arteries cannot supply the heart with enough blood to meet the extra demands of the task in hand but sometimes it is caused by an actual reduction in blood supply, probably the result of arterial *spasm* (see explanations). This narrows the arteries and is probably the cause of some kinds of angina, particularly of angina at rest. For practical purposes angina however produced can be assumed to be associated with coronary artery disease.

The clinical feature of angina is pain in the centre of

the chest occurring during the course of exercise or exertion. The pain is more a sense of pressure under the breast bone and even of strangulation as the Greek word for angina (ankoné) implies. It is often mistaken for severe indigestion. Pain is also likely to be felt in other parts of the body which share the same nerve supply as the heart. These are the arms, the neck, the upper part of the back and the jaw. Sometimes this distant pain (referred pain) is more prominent than the chest pain and is misinterpreted as "rheumatism". Quite often, too, people consult a dentist in the belief that they have toothache. The true nature of the pain can generally be recognised by its constant relationship to exercise which it nearly always interrupts and by its tendency to become localised to a single point such as the bend of the elbow or the wrist. People have even removed a bangle or a wrist watch in an attempt to stop it.

The amount of exercise a person with angina can take remains relatively constant for the individual but is not directly related to the extent of the underlying disease. Some with severe arterial damage are relatively, or for a time even totally, free from angina, others with minor damage are seriously affected. Generally however angina is slowly progressive over a long time. At first it may occur only during strenuous exertion such as sprinting for a bus or running upstairs. Later it can come on during quick walking uphill. Eventually it occurs with gradually decreasing effort until it can virtually prohibit any effective physical activity. Characteristically people with angina may be seen walking along steadily but stopping periodically, perhaps ostensibly to look into a shop window, to gain relief before going on. Feelings of emotion such as anger may precipitate angina. It is nearly always worse in cold weather as well as after a meal which provokes additional activity by the heart. Angina begins to go off as soon as the stimulus which has provoked it is reduced or removed and seldom lasts more than five minutes or at the most a quarter of an hour. Pain lasting longer is likely to be a sign of more permanent damage to the heart muscle, such as a "coronary". Though years often pass without any noticeable worsening, angina can be complicated by a coronary which can alter its course. Sudden death, although unusual, can occur in an attack especially if physical exertion is continued.

A variant of classical angina pectoris (thought to be due to spasm, see page 87) has attracted considerable attention since the pain though in other ways characteristic comes when the person is sitting quietly or resting. Such people may also suffer from angina of effort but sometimes do not. Another less common phenomenon is so called "warm up angina" in which pain is provoked when exercise is first undertaken but then passes off so that subsequent exercise can be taken without pain.

The treatment of angina

Angina may be provoked by diseases such as severe anaemia, and thyroid gland deficiency (myxoedema), and also by heavy cigarette smoking. They should always be looked for. Although coronary artery disease may be present as well their successful treatment and/or the cutting out of smoking cigarettes will nearly always improve the angina and sometimes appears to cure it. Other diseases of the heart and circulation such as aortic valve disease (Chapter 2), or high blood pressure should also be identified and dealt with appropriately if they are present. Otherwise treatment should attempt to improve the performance of the heart. Weight reduction where necessary will often help but drugs which interfere with some of the actions of adrenaline (propranolol equals inderal) and glyceryl trinitrate, which reduces the work of the heart by dilating the resistance arteries, are invaluable. Both drugs enable the heart to do more work without pain.

Adrenaline antagonists act gradually but last for some hours. Tablets should be taken four times daily in the quantity directed. Long acting preparations of nitrates are available and can be taken in the same way but glyceryl trinitrate itself acts immediately and lasts for a matter of minutes. It should therefore be carried conveniently ready for instant use when the occasion arises. To get the best from it a tablet should be placed under the tongue before beginning any activity likely to cause angina. Glyceryl trinitrate may cause headaches particularly when first used but they are not generally severe enough to limit its value.

If an attack of angina begins physical activity *must stop* until the pain has gone completely. "Sit down if you can but stand still if you cannot" is the absolute rule. To go on is dangerous. Glyceryl trinitrate taken as soon as an attack seems to be coming can sometimes abort it. Later on it probably has little effect. Provided that the rule of stopping activity during an attack is obeyed exercise does nothing but good. If angina fails to improve with these measures surgical treatment should be considered (see later, page 133).

Coronary thrombosis: a "coronary"

A "coronary" is a popular term for a clinical event brought about by sudden or nearly sudden damage to the heart muscle. The underlying cause is nearly always obstruction by thrombosis of a branch of a coronary artery which may be either previously healthy or the site of pre-existing disease. An alternative view that arterial spasm (see explanations) often initiates the coronary obstruction has been put forward to explain the apparent absence of thrombosis in some fatal cases. Further evidence is needed to support it.

The area of heart muscle supplied by the affected artery is deprived of blood and in due course dies. This leaves a permanent scar. The process is known as infarction. In the expectation that the damage to the heart muscle has been caused by arterial obstruction by a thrombosis doctors often speak of a "coronary" as a coronary thrombosis. Since there is no direct proof of thrombosis in an artery this diagnosis is an assumption although a very likely one. For this reason a diagnosis of "myocardial infarction" which refers to the probable nature of the muscle damage is sometimes preferred.

Clinical features of coronary thrombosis

The outstanding feature of a "coronary" is pain similar in situation, distribution and character to that of angina. But since the pain of a coronary is caused by permanent muscle damage it lasts longer than the pain of angina which is caused by a temporary failure of the heart's blood supply. Usually it lasts for some hours although exceptionally it may continue for one or two days before finally ceasing. As explained elsewhere a coronary generally occurs at rest with the person sitting quietly or even lying down whereas angina generally occurs during exercise. Less often it begins during exercise like an attack of angina but then instead of being shortlived when the exercise stops, continues. Occasionally a coronary shows itself as repeated attacks of angina occurring after shorter and shorter periods of activity and sometimes also occurring at rest during the course of a few days or a week. This is known as "crescendo angina".

A coronary sometimes begins in an unusual way, even without pain. The sudden onset of heart failure (see page 65) or of a serious disorder of the heart beat in a previously healthy person are events which should at least raise a suspicion of a coronary. Other symptoms such as faintness or loss of consciousness caused by a sudden reduction in the circulation to the brain sometimes suggest that a stroke is impending. Occasionally there are convulsions not unlike those of an epileptic fit.

The muscle damage occurring with a coronary usually weakens the pumping power of the heart. This may be severe enough to cause shock if the output of blood falls drastically and the blood pressure drops sharply. In very severe cases the circulation to the brain and to the heart itself will suffer and may even fail completely. The patient then loses consciousness and dies. More often the effects are less grave and reduce quickly causing only a feeling of faintness sometimes accompanied by brief loss of consciousness and by vomiting. Compensatory narrowing of the smaller arteries in the body (vaso-constriction) follows and diverts blood from the skin and the muscles to protect the circulation to vital parts of the body such as the brain, the kidneys and the heart itself. The patient feels weak and sweats, the limbs become cold and the skin pale until recovery takes place.

The twenty four hours following a coronary are a period of danger. Even if shock is absent disorders of the heart beat are common and, together sometimes with varying degrees of heart block (see Chapter 3) caused by damage to the conducting system, may further weaken the heart's action. The first two or three hours are a time of great danger when serious disturbances of the heart beat such as ventricular tachycardia and ventricular fibrillation are liable to occur and are likely to be fatal unless promptly treated (see Chapter 7). The danger lessens progressively and the circulation generally recovers. A day or two or at the most a week are usually enough to enable the patient to move about in bed and to begin to do things for himself. Sometimes where there is a degree of heart failure, or there are persistent conduction defects or irregularities of the heart beat, continued or even prolonged treatment may be needed but most cases recover early. The muscle damage needs a month or more to heal.

In uncomplicated cases recovery aided by physical and mental rehabilitation can be virtually complete. The patient should be able to return to full activity after about three months. With suitable training and medical advice many people can progressively resume normal physical activity sometimes including fairly vigorous sport.

As mentioned complications such as chronic heart failure, persistent defects of conduction and irregularities of the heart beat may hinder recovery in the early stages and will need appropriate treatment. A number of factors, particularly the extent of the damage may also influence the long term outlook. For example older people and those with previous heart damage or high blood pressure tend to fare worse. However, even in them, correction of obesity, giving up cigarette smoking and reorganising an unsatisfactory life-style may improve the outlook and help to prevent further attacks.

Recognition of a coronary thrombosis

The clinical features just described generally justify a presumptive diagnosis of a coronary by themselves. Proof comes from unequivocal evidence of characteristic damage to the heart muscle.

This is usually provided by finding chemical changes in the blood and by abnormalities recorded in the electrocardiogram, or by both. The chemical events in contracting muscle depend upon the release of energy by the action of enzymes. Damage to muscle and especially heart muscle releases these enzymes temporarily into the blood. Some of them exist only in heart muscle and the levels which they reach in the blood give some idea of the extent of the damage and of the time when it has occurred. They are particularly valuable in the diagnosis of muscle damage which, either because of its location, or because it is very limited in extent, may escape recognition by electrocardiography. However the electrocardiogram provides the most reliable evidence of the site and the extent of muscle damage.

Immediately after a coronary the part of the heart muscle affected is injured but not dead. Injured muscle of this kind is at a different electrical potential from normal resting muscle. Current therefore flows between resting muscle and recently damaged muscle and distorts the electrocardiogram. This current which is known as the current of injury, lasts until the injured muscle dies and becomes electrically inactive. Afterwards evidence of permanent loss of muscle appears and shows itself by reduction of the normal electrical activity of contraction (depolarisation) at the site of the damage and by an alteration in the direction of the recovery process (repolarisation).

Fig. 10 shows the progressive electrocardiographic changes in the damaged area and should be compared with Fig. 6 which depicts the normal state prior to a coronary. The detailed significance of the letters P. Q. R. S. T. is explained on page 114.

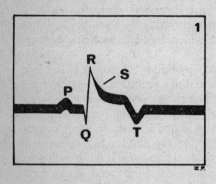

SOON AFTER CORONARY THROMBOSIS

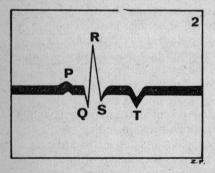

LATE STAGE

Fig. 10 Electrocardiogram: Showing effects of coronary thrombosis.
1. Current of injury. Shown by upward deflection of the S.T. segment at end of ventricular contraction.
2. Permanent damage. S.T. segment no longer elevated. T. permanently inverted.

Treatment of a "coronary"

Immediate treatment (see also emergency treatment, page 129). A coronary is a medical emergency. The first thing is to prevent shock. The patient must be kept warm and pain must be relieved as soon as possible by suitable drugs. Morphine or a similar drug is generally needed. Complete rest is imperative until the heart is again working normally.

Circulatory failure, irregularities of the heart beat, and conduction defects which often accompany or follow a coronary, are potentially recoverable provided that they are diagnosed and treated immediately. A coronary occurring in hospital or in a patient admitted to hospital is therefore best treated in a special ward which is equipped to monitor the heart's action by continuous electrocardiography. Everything needed to correct disorders of the heart beat and if necessary to resuscitate the patient if the heart stops should be available. Wards of this kind need expensive equipment and highly trained staff. They have been criticised as unnecessary and potentially harmful, but there is clear evidence that patients suffering a coronary when already in hospital fare much better in them than those in ordinary wards. Reductions in mortality from more than 30% to less than 10% have been achieved sufficiently often to justify them.

The proper management for patients who suffer a coronary outside hospital – the majority – is not so easy to decide. If the illness occurs at home there is often considerable delay in notifying a doctor and in obtaining medical attention. Provided he can be properly looked after, it may be preferable to leave the patient where he is rather than subject him to the physical and psychological upset of transfer to hospital by ambulance. Some large scale surveys seem to favour this course but better provision of special ambulance services equipped to deal with emergencies and organised to go promptly to any suspected "coronary" may alter the situation.

A patient suffering a coronary in the street or away from home should be taken to hospital at once, preferably in an ambulance equipped to give emergency treatment on the way. Prompt action by a well informed bystander may serve whilst it is coming (see Chapter 7 page 130). What really counts is the length of time before a person receives competent treatment. Within the first three or four hours the potential danger from treatable and even preventable disturbances of the heart beat justifies any possible risk of transfer to hospital. Afterwards the immediate benefits are less. Once the initial period of danger is over, the decision must be taken on other grounds.

Further treatment

For many years patients were kept in bed for about a month after a "coronary" in the belief that this would allow time for the damaged muscle to heal. This prolonged immobility was quite unnecessary and only encouraged thrombosis in the deep veins of the body and lower limbs with the consequent risk of pulmonary embolism (see Chapter 3.) Patients are now allowed out of bed as soon as their heart is working normally and leave hospital after a week or at the most ten days provided that they are free from complications such as any important degree of heart failure, conduction defects or persistent disorders of the heart beat. Once out of bed convalescence with graduated activity begins.

Standing, washing and dressing, at first under supervision, prepare for the return home. At first a ground floor bed is advisable but afterwards walking in the garden, climbing stairs slowly and undertaking easy domestic tasks should lead to a gradual resumption of normal home life within a month. Later other activities such as car driving (subject to medical advice – also check your insurance) may follow with the aim of a return to work at the end of two to three months. Convalescence is often a period of frustration, depression and anxiety and the patient needs constant encouragement.

Once past the initial phase patients must learn to regulate their own activities. Special diets are unnecessary but those who are overweight should reduce gradually and heavy cigarette smoking should be cut. The only bars on physical activity, other than sudden activities such as sprinting and static exercise such as pushing a stationary car, which are always dangerous, are angina and breathlessness.

The particular characteristics of angina can be learned by the patient and his relatives by reference to the initial coronary pain. It must be distinguished clearly from other symptoms some of which can be ignored. For instance some people after a coronary become particularly aware of their heart beat. They notice a quicker and more forcible heart beat when first getting up and about. Provided that this is not accompanied by breathlessness or the pain of angina and provided that it is not fast enough or irregular enough to suggest a major disorder of the heart beat (Chapter 3) it can be ignored. It will improve with activity. Others experience a dull ache in the left side of the chest of which the cause is uncertain. Both problems are often a source of unnecessary anxiety but are not dangerous and should be disregarded. True angina is always a signal to stop whatever is being done until it has passed off. Those who have suffered from angina before a coronary sometimes lose it afterwards. Others may acquire it for the first time. Angina occurring after a coronary should be treated on the lines already described.

The amount of physical exercise which can be undertaken after a coronary depends largely upon the patient's general condition. Those who are old or infirm and those who have never taken vigorous exercise should not attempt to exceed their normal level of activity. Others can eventually often regain physical fitness for sport and even return to long distance running on their doctor's advice. Supervision in a gymnasium where graduated exercise on a fixed bicycle is possible and where other standards of fitness can be measured is both physically and mentally helpful.

As soon as possible a coronary should be treated as a

finished event except for the need to visit the doctor periodically. All the emphasis should be on sensible progress and not on restriction. The risks of recurrence are greatest during the first year and particularly during the first six months after the initial attack. Drugs which interfere with blood clotting, are sometimes used in the early stages of the illness. In the longer term aspirin when carefully prescribed, may lessen the risk of recurrence. After the first year this diminishes progressively until after about ten years life expectancy is equal to that of healthy people of the same age. Anti-adrenaline drugs, e.g. propranolol, will diminish the risks.

SURGERY FOR CORONARY HEART DISEASE

Until recently the pattern of heart muscle damage shown on an electrocardiogram provided the only evidence of the extent and distribution of the underlying arterial disease. Injection directly into the coronary arteries of opaque dye which can be visualised by suitable X-Rays (coronary angiography) makes possible more exact and in many cases remarkably accurate assessment of their state. This has greatly improved the prospects for more radical treatment by surgery. Various procedures have been devised but the most satisfactory at present is bypass of part of the diseased artery by a graft taken from a vein in the leg. Neither the operation nor the preliminary X-Ray examination are entirely free from risk so that they should not be undertaken unless the limitations imposed by angina are severe and have failed to improve with simpler measures and with drug treatment. Above all they should be carried out only by those specially experienced in the work. It is perhaps too early to evaluate the long term place for surgery but short term results are enormously encouraging. Only a few patients find such an operation fails to improve things and there is increasing evidence that in severe cases the prospects for life may also be better.

5
HIGH BLOOD PRESSURE (HYPERTENSION)

"High blood pressure" often spoken of as "hypertension" refers to the systemic circulation. It means that the pressure exerted by the blood in the aorta and its branches persistently exceeds the upper limits of normal. Normal limits have been derived from mean figures taken from large numbers of healthy people. As indicated in Chapter 1 pressures are measured in millimetres of mercury (mmHg.) and two measurements are made. They are the systolic pressure with a normal level of 140 mmHg. and the diastolic pressure, normally about 90 mmHg. as recorded in a person lying or sitting down quietly. Pressures vary considerably in healthy people. Systolic levels between 90–150 mmHg. and diastolic levels between 60–90 mmHg. are not unusual. There is a tendency for pressures to rise with age and pressures of 160/100 mmHg. are generally accepted as normal in people aged 60 and older.

There are a number of reasons why blood pressure levels vary widely in health. For one thing the standard method of measurement is not precise and is open to errors of observation and to errors dependent upon the thickness of the subject's arm. To allow for this readings are generally taken to the nearest one to two millimetre point. Also the regulation of the blood pressure is complex and depends both on the output of the heart and on the resistance set up in the circulation by the smaller arteries (peripheral resistance). The peripheral resistance is the more important and particularly affects the diastolic pressure. When the peripheral resistance is increased the blood pressure tends to rise unless the output of the heart is appreciably reduced. When it is lowered it often prevents the blood pressure from rising even when the output of the heart is considerably raised.

Both the output of the heart and the peripheral resistance are influenced by a number of bodily processes and particularly by the action of the sympathetic nervous system, the secretion of adrenaline and noradrenaline by the suprarenal glands and the regulation of the blood volume by the kidneys. These in turn react sensitively to a number of biological situations which in this way become responsible for temporary changes in blood pressure. For example, when people stand up more blood is held in the veins under the influence of gravity. Less is therefore returned to the heart and the output of the heart is temporarily reduced. On the other hand the peripheral resistance tends to be increased. Consequently overall the systolic pressure may fall by up to 10 mmHg. and the diastolic pressure may rise by up to 5 mmHg. Feelings of emotion, extra mental activity such as when doing arithmetic, some forms of physical exertion including sexual intercourse, and exposure to cold are all liable to increase the peripheral resistance and sometimes the heart's output and therefore to raise the blood pressure. More prolonged situations such as an overacting thyroid gland or states of continuing anxiety can raise the heart's output persistently and raise the systolic pressure. Drugs, such as oral contraceptives, "adrenal steroids" and some pain killers, increase the blood volume by causing sodium to be retained in the body and thus raise the output of the heart. All of them may provoke small or even appreciable rises of blood pressure which usually disappear when the cause is removed. In contrast the increased output of the heart which is a feature particularly of pregnancy and of severe anaemia is usually accompanied by a lowered arterial resistance. When this happens the blood pressure does not rise and may even fall.

Clearly a number of factors have to be taken into account when interpreting blood pressure readings. A diagnosis of "hypertension" should seldom be made solely on the evidence of a single reading.

CAUSES OF HYPERTENSION

Secondary hypertension

Disease affecting parts of the body other than the heart and circulatory system can cause hypertension although the way in which it does so is not always understood. Hypertension occurring in these circumstances is known as secondary hypertension. Various forms of kidney disease provide the commonest examples. Less common but equally important because they can often be successfully treated, are congenital narrowing of the aorta (coarctation, see Chapter 2) and overactivity of the pituitary or of the suprarenal glands which is sometimes associated with tumour formation.

Kidney disease is of special interest because the kidneys are known to secrete a substance (renin) which after enzymatic transformation is able to raise the blood pressure. Secondary hypertension affects the heart and blood vessels in the same way as essential hypertension. The other characteristic features of these underlying diseases are beyond the scope of this book, however they must be looked for in every case of hypertension in order that secondary hypertension can be discovered or ruled out.

Essential hypertension

The commonest form of hypertension is essential hypertension in which as the name implies there is no evidence of structural disease in any organ other than the heart and blood vessels. No single cause for it has yet been identified but both main regulators of the blood pressure seem to be implicated. In the early stages of the disease the high blood pressure is often associated with a raised output of the heart, possibly the result of overaction of the sympathetic nervous system. Once the disease has become established the heart's output generally becomes normal and an increased peripheral resistance maintains the high blood pressure. Although there are no signs of structural disease in the kidneys it is possible and indeed likely that a disorder of kidney function and in particular a failure to handle sodium and so to control the circulating blood volume has a rôle in essential hypertension.

Whatever the underlying mechanism a constitutional liability to generate particularly high pressure in face of a variety of stimuli seems to be also partly responsible. For example people who produce exceptionally high pressures when exposed to cold are eventually likely to develop hypertension. Again sufferers from migraine, a disorder of the arteries to the brain, often become hypertensive in middle life. Both findings support the view that "hypertensives" have unusually sensitive resistance arteries and are more likely than normal people to develop high, and perhaps very high, pressures in response to the ups and downs of everyday life. Repeated temporary rises of pressure in such people eventually produce structural changes in the smaller arteries which permanently increase the peripheral resistance and so perpetuate the hypertension.

The constitutional tendency in hypertensive people is partly familial and probably genetic since those with one hypertensive parent are more likely, and those with two hypertensive parents much more likely, to develop hypertension. Environmental and acquired factors however reinforce the tendency and do much to determine the severity of the disease. The greatest prevalence of essential hypertension seems to be in affluent "Westernised" societies whilst others are relatively immune. It is particularly uncommon in rural African societies but urbanised Africans develop hypertension as easily and sometimes more severely than Europeans. Features of these urbanised societies which have been blamed are obesity and a high intake of salt in the diet, but emotional tension and a stressful life style are usually given pride of place.

The importance of obesity is supported by the finding that weight reduction by dieting sometimes seems to reduce the blood pressure. A possible explanation is that a lower intake of food reduces metabolism and lowers the turnover of substances such as adrenaline and noradrenaline. A high intake of salt may increase the blood volume. Reduction to almost negligible levels on the other hand can sometimes lower the blood pressure. This kind of treatment however is often unacceptable in practice and has indeed been challenged on the ground that the amount of potassium in food is at least as important as salt (sodium).

Personality is always difficult to evaluate. Although many hypertensives seem normal enough a proportion are undoubtedly emotionally tense. Sufferers from psychological disease characterised by extreme changes of mood (manic/depressive disorders) may be liable to experience fluctuations in blood pressure with low pressures in periods of depression and high pressure in periods of elation. The mood changes may be severe enough to interfere seriously with the treatment of hypertension. Relief of physical and mental tension by rest and sedation in the early stages of hypertension, will sometimes lower high blood pressures even to normal levels. Such relief however is nearly always short lived. The high pressures return when, as so often happens, the patient returns to his former way of life, unless he is able to reform the personality traits responsible.

All in all essential hypertension seems likely to occur when people with a constitutional tendency to react hypertensively to a wide range of stimuli are exposed to a "stressful environment" and to particular habits of life. The tendency is probably not a simple "either or" reaction but a liability varying with the individual's constitution and with the severity of the conditions to which he is exposed, or to which he exposes himself.

THE COURSE OF HYPERTENSION

Essential hypertension is generally first discovered between the ages of 40 and 60 but is sometimes found much earlier. Men and women are equally likely to be affected. Two kinds are recognised: benign and accelerated, the latter sometimes called malignant.

Benign hypertension

As a rule the blood pressure is initially moderately and sometimes only intermittently raised. Pressures at first of the order of 180/100, rise progressively but gradually to levels around 240/130. The rate of increase is variable and may spread over a period from five to 15 years. This slowly progressive character delays the onset of damage to the heart and blood vessels and is responsible for the term "benign" which is used to describe the usual form of the disease and distinguish it from the more rapidly progressive but rarer "malignant" (accelerated) form. Benign hypertension is often symptomless in its early stages and may only be detected during a routine medical examination. Those who are naturally prone to headaches sometimes complain of a dull ache at the back of the head or of a throbbing sensation which may be accompanied by giddiness at the top of the head. Others notice more forcible beating of the heart.

Accelerated hypertension

Accelerated hypertension affects a few "hypertensives". It is characterised by exceptionally high pressures and by a more rapid rise of pressure. Consequently the damage to the heart and arteries occurs sooner and is more severe than in benign hypertension. Damage to the small arteries of the kidneys is almost inevitable.

Accelerated hypertension sometimes raises the pressure within the skull. This causes headaches at the back which are usually worse when people lie down. They are consequently likely to occur on first waking especially at weekends when many people allow themselves a longer lie in.

In the long run the only indisputable symptoms of hypertension are caused by damage to the heart and arteries. The severity of hypertension depends upon the amount of damage to them. This varies from person to person and depends partly upon the height and consistency of the raised pressure, partly upon the constitutional strength of the individual and partly upon the life he leads. Women generally fare better than men.

THE EFFECTS OF HYPERTENSION

Some people seem relatively unaffected and enjoy a normal life span. The majority run into trouble after a period of years. Accelerated hypertension untreated lasts for about two years. Fortunately treatment is usually successful.

Damage to the heart: Hypertensive heart disease

A persistently high systemic arterial pressure causes hypertensive heart disease. High systolic pressures and or high diastolic pressures almost always cause trouble. The extra pressures impose a strain on the left ventricle which at first generally hypertrophies and manages to maintain an effective circulation against the increased resistance. However eventually the muscle weakens, dilation of the ventricle follows and the heart begins to fail. Since the extra strain of hypertension falls entirely upon the left ventricle, left ventricular failure with cardiac asthma (see Chapter 3) may be the first sign of heart failure.

Damage to the coronary arteries is not uncommon and sometimes leads to angina or to coronary thrombosis. This may hasten the onset of heart failure (see page 68), particularly if coronary thrombosis occurs.

Damage to the arteries

Arterial damage chiefly affects the small and medium sized arteries such as those to the brain and the kidneys. Damage to the arteries of the brain may result in a stroke following either obstruction by thrombosis or rupture with bleeding into the substance of the brain. A stroke comes on suddenly and usually causes loss of consciousness followed by loss of function of the damaged area of the brain. According to the site of the damage this may show itself as paralysis of one side of the body or of a single part such as the face, an arm or a leg. Paralysis is sometimes accompanied by impaired vision, and if it affects the right side of the body, defective speech. A stroke caused by thrombosis may recover to some extent but bleeding of any severity into the brain tends to be progressive and is likely to be fatal. Temporary disorders such as brief loss of vision or speech or partial paralysis can be caused by temporary disturbances of the circulation to the brain and may precede a stroke.

High blood pressure also affects the arteries to the kidneys. In the case of benign hypertension the damage is generally unimportant and the kidneys continue to function normally. Accelerated hypertension causes much more serious damage and generally leads to kidney failure unless it is effectively treated. This is one of the most serious consequences of the disease. The narrowing and irregularity in small arteries caused by high blood pressure affects the arteries at the back of the eye (retinal arteries). They can be seen with a suitable instrument and give a fair picture of the extent of damage to the smaller arteries in other parts of the body, and therefore a reasonably accurate indication of the severity of the disease. Disturbances of vision occur fairly often in accelerated hypertension but are less common in benign hypertension.

RECOGNITION OF HYPERTENSION

As indicated earlier, warning symptoms are difficult to interpret and the only certain way of recognising hypertension is by taking the blood pressure. Large scale screening of populations is being advocated and is becoming practicable but is unlikely to become universal in the immediate future. Recognition in individuals likely to be affected is therefore important. People over 30 seeing a doctor for the first time should always have their blood pressure taken. Those with a family history should make a point of doing so and may be advised to have periodical examinations afterwards. Sufferers from migraine, and women who have had high blood pressure during pregnancy, are others particularly at risk.

TREATMENT OF HYPERTENSION

The improved prospects for treating hypertension and of averting the damaging consequences just described are largely the result of the introduction of a whole range of drugs. Provided that they are recognised before the heart and arteries have been seriously damaged, most cases can be treated successfully. When damage to the heart and arteries has already occurred treatment is vitally necessary. It will help to prevent further damage and in some cases will reverse existing damage. Accelerated hypertension responds particularly well unless irreversible changes have occurred in the kidneys. Even then the possibility of maintaining kidney function by artificial kidneys and the increasing availability of kidney transplants mark an important step forward.

A number of remedies for hypertension have been devised. None of them cures the disease since the hypertensive tendency is always present. Treatment must therefore be continued and lifelong. At one time operations were performed to lessen nervous influences on the blood pressure by removing portions of the sympathetic nervous system. Subsequently they were replaced by drugs designed to interfere chemically with the action of adrenaline and noradrenaline on the smaller arteries and so to lower the peripheral resistance in the circulation.

Inevitably these drugs affect the normal adjustments of the circulation, particularly the responses to exercise and to changes of posture. Consequently when such drugs are used falls in pressure which may be severe enough to cause fainting sometimes occur with strenuous exercise – and when standing up quickly after lying down, particularly when getting up in the morning. Newer drugs and careful regulation of dosage, however, have gone some way to overcome these unwanted effects and to produce steadier levels of blood pressure.

Another approach uses diuretics to stimulate the excretion of salt and water by the kidneys. Both kinds of treatment can be used together.

The success of drug treatment should not divert attention from the possibilities of a more fundamental approach to the management of hypertension. Every case must be carefully examined to ensure that there is no underlying cause such as a congenital narrowing of the aorta, or a secreting tumour of either the pituitary or supra-renal gland, or even a diseased kidney on one side which can be removed. Reduction of weight in those who are obese will often lower the blood pressure. Drastic reduction of the intake of salt can be helpful if it is acceptable. Cigarette smoking, though perhaps not directly responsible for the disease, can be given up with advantage. Various methods of reducing psychological and physical tensions ranging from the use of tranquillising drugs to relaxation therapy, yoga, and deep meditation have their advocates. All have some success to their credit but all of them in the long run probably need to be supplemented by appropriate drug treatment.

Apart from the need to produce more acceptable preparations the main problems of drug treatment are how to detect the disease in the early stages, when to begin treatment and how to ensure that it is continued effectively.

The decision to begin treatment is always difficult. High pressures in those under 40, a diastolic pressure persistently above 100 mmHg., or signs of damage to the heart, the arteries or the kidneys are clear cut indications. Malignant hypertension demands immediate and carefully controlled treatment which should usually begin in hospital. With lower pressures and in the absence of signs in the heart and arteries it is possible to await developments and many physicians prefer to advise measures designed to correct an obviously faulty way of living before submitting patients to a lifelong regime which is not without disadvantages and even dangers. The value of treatment in the elderly is debatable. Very high pressures, particularly diastolic pressures, should probably be reduced at any age but levels a little above normal are best left alone and may even be beneficial at an advanced age.

Treatment once begun must be regularly maintained and controlled. Although the introduction of instruments which enable patients to record their own blood pressure promises to be helpful, periodic visits to a doctor are bound to be necessary to ensure that drugs are being correctly taken and that there are no signs of any complications of the disease or of unwanted effects of treatment. Once instituted treatment should practically never be abandoned. Interruption of treatment can cause a sudden swing back to high and even very high levels of pressure with potentially serious risks.

6
HOW HEART DISEASE IS DISCOVERED

Paradoxically the majority of those going to a doctor because they think they have heart disease are mistaken. On the other hand significant symptoms such as the pain of Angina or the breathlessness of early heart failure (see page 65), which a doctor would recognise fairly easily, are often ignored or misinterpreted. A full description (history) of a person's symptoms is essential and often gives a doctor a clear picture of what is wrong even before he has made his examination. The most important symptoms have been described earlier (Chapter 3).

Increasing breathlessness on exertion is the most important indication that the heart is beginning to fail. Sometimes it is accompanied by breathlessness when lying down and less often by the severe breathlessness of Cardiac Asthma (see page 68). It may be preceded by tiredness or faintness on exertion sometimes accompanied by coldness and aching of the legs. These are symptoms of many diseases and it is the breathlessness which is important. Palpitation may draw attention to disorders of the heart beat. The rapid and sometimes irregular beating of major disorders such as atrial fibrillation and atrial flutter can usually be felt in the chest and sometimes accurately described. Minor disorders such as ectopic beats are sometimes noticed as "a jump" in the chest or as a double heart beat. Sudden loss of consciousness may indicate the presence of Complete Heart Block. The characteristic features of a "coronary" are often the first indication of coronary heart disease but people sometimes notice Angina Pectoris before this. Heart disease can also be symptomless. Congenital malformations and valvular disease are often first detected by chance medical examination.

PHYSICAL EXAMINATIONS

Physical examinations can tell a doctor a lot about the state of the heart and the circulation. Heart failure for instance usually produces characteristic signs. Congestion of the lungs caused by left heart failure can often be detected by listening to the chest. A raised pressure in the systemic veins caused by right heart failure shows itself by distension and pulsation of the deep veins in the neck. Enlargement of the liver and dropsy in the lower back or the legs can readily be found by appropriate examination. Feeling the heart through the chest wall (palpation) will often identify irregularities of the heart beat and may also enable a doctor to discover enlargement (dilatation or hypertrophy) of either ventricle. Abnormal closure of the heart valves tends to produce characteristic sounds which can be heard with a stethoscope and abnormal blood flow through the valves

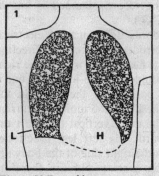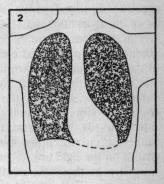

Fig. 11 X-Ray of heart.
1. Heart enlarged by muscle disease.
2. Normal size after recovery.
   Key: H = Heart.
            L = Lung.

produces high frequency sounds known as murmurs which can generally be detected and fairly accurately interpreted in this way. The arterial pulse gives additional information about the rate and regularity of the heart beat, but is often equally valuable as an indication of the volume and character of the output of the left ventricle. It is therefore useful in estimating the severity of valvular disease. Simple X-Rays of the chest will estimate the size of the heart and the extent and location of any enlargement fairly accurately.

Electrocardiography

The electrocardiograph is an instrument designed to record the size and direction of the electrical current transmitted through the body when the heart beats. The basic principles of this flow of current were described in Chapter 1. A number of systems of measurement have been devised but essentially all consist of a galvanometer, calibrated to give a deflection of one millimetre for differences of electrical potential of one millivolt, a time marker and a recording mechanism. The last is a lever, usually a hot wire, which moves with the galvanometer and writes on specially sensitised paper. The record obtained is known as an electrocardiogram (E.C.G.).

The electrocardiograph records differences of electrical potential between paired electrodes. The general direction of the flow of current when the heart beats is from the right shoulder towards the left shoulder or the left foot, but it varies appreciably with the position of the heart in the chest. The more horizontal the heart the more the current flows towards the left arm, the more vertical the heart the more the current flows towards the left leg. Electrodes placed on the right arm or on the right side of the body are normally in the wake of the current and are therefore electrically negative in relation to electrodes placed on the left arm, the left leg or the left side of the body which face the approaching current. The recording mechanism is arranged so that an upward deflection from the base line records electrically positive changes, and a downward deflection records electrically negative changes.

The first type of electrocardiogram which was ever recorded is known as the standard electrocardiogram. It is still used and is a record of potential differences between three separate pairs of electrodes. The combinations are known as leads. Lead I records the difference between the right arm and the left arm. Lead II the difference between the right arm and the left leg and Lead III the difference between the left arm and the left leg.

The standard electrocardiogram is limited in several ways. The electrodes are relatively distant from the heart and therefore record only a general picture of its electrical activity. They also record activity only in the frontal plane of the body. The standard electrocardiogram therefore needs to be supplemented by records taken from electrodes placed on the chest directly over the heart (chest leads). These record current flowing at right angles to the body surface and also, being closer to the heart, give a more detailed picture of the electrical activity at the site of each electrode. (Refer to Fig. 12). Chest leads are recorded from six positions, starting from position one (1) on the right of the breast bone and crossing to the left with position six (6) on the chest wall below the left arm. Chest electrodes may be paired with an electrode on the right arm and are known as C.R. leads (1–6). Less often they are paired with an electrode on the left foot (C.F. leads).

Standard electrocardiograms and chest leads of the kind described, however, record only differences of potential between opposite sides of the body and do not measure directly the changes transmitted to each electrode. To overcome this on the standard electrocardiogram each electrode on the body is paired with a central terminal which thus finds itself connected to all three limb electrodes. This has a zero potential and enables the actual voltage changes occurring at each electrode on the body to be measured. Leads of this kind are "voltage" or V. leads and the changes they record are small in comparison with those recorded by standard and other leads so they need to be augmented artificially. They are therefore known as a V. leads, the left arm being, a VL., the left foot, a VF., and the right arm, a VR. Chest "voltage" leads taken in this way are known as V_{1-6}.

A normal standard electrocardiogram has five main deflections from the base line (see Fig. 6). They are arbitrarily designated by five consecutive letters of the alphabet P.Q.R.S.T. The P. wave represents the electrical activity when the two atria contract. Q.R.S. represent the electrical activity of the various phases of ventricular contraction; and T. represents the recovery activity of the ventricles. The interval between the first upward deflection of P. and the first deflection of Q.R.S. (either Q. or R. when Q. is very small) represents the time taken for the excitation process to spread from the atria to the ventricles and is therefore a measure of conduction from atria to ventricles. It should not exceed 0.2 (1/5) secs. It is prolonged in heart block. The width of Q.R.S. represents the time taken by contraction of both ventricles and should not exceed 0.1 (1/10) secs. Q.R.S. taking longer than 0.1 sec. probably indicates delay of conduction to one ventricle (Bundle Branch Block, see Chapter 3).

Standard electrocardiograms principally show upward deflections in all leads indicating the predominant effect of the current approaching the left arm and the left leg. The flow of current to the left arm is similar in magnitude to the flow to the left leg. The deflections of Lead III which represent the potential differences between the left arm electrode and the left leg electrode are therefore generally smaller particularly in the Q.R.S.T. wave than those for Leads I and II. a V leads show that the potential recorded at the right arm is electrically negative (downwards deflection) throughout the ventricular part of the heart beat but the left arm and the left foot leads are positive (upward deflection). Chest leads from the right side are similar to those in the right arm but progressively approximate to those in the left arm as they cross the body from right to left.

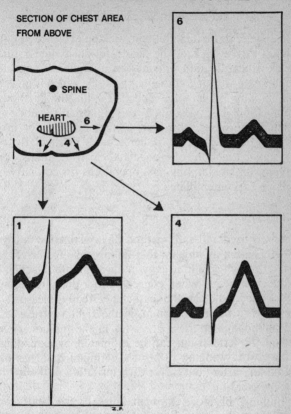

Fig. 12 Normal chest leads taken in positions 1, 4 and 6 on chest.

When the left ventricle hypertrophies the direction of the heart's electrical activity moves towards the left arm, when the right ventricle hypertrophies it moves towards the left leg. The electrocardiogram may therefore reveal valuable information about the state of the ventricles. For its uses in other conditions, see Chapters 3 and 4.

OTHER INVESTIGATIONS

In spite of its limited ability to pick up evidence of muscle damage at the back of the heart and on its under surface the electrocardiogram provides an indispensable record of the intimate working of the heart muscle which is unobtainable in any other way. Together with the methods of examination just described this is usually enough for practical purposes. However, further methods of investigation are available in difficult cases particularly when surgical correction of congenital malformations, or of valvular disease, and by-pass operations for coronary heart disease, are contemplated.

Catheterisation

A well tried and safe method of investigation is cardiac catheterisation in which a thin hollow tube (catheter) is inserted through a vein, usually in the arm, into the chambers of the right heart. When connected to a pressure recording device (manometer) the catheter directly measures the pressures in the right atrium, in the right ventricle and in the pulmonary arteries. Pressures in the pulmonary veins and in the left atrium can be estimated by extending the catheter and wedging it into the terminal branches of the pulmonary artery but direct catheterisation of the left heart is more usual.

Shunting of blood through holes in the heart can be detected and measured by estimating the oxygen content of blood in different chambers. Excess oxygenation of the blood in the right heart will indicate a left to right shunt.

Contrast Radiography

Injection of substances which can be visualised by X-Rays and of radio active material which can be visualised by suitable scanning devices has also proved useful in defining the shape, size and contractile force of individual chambers of the heart, but perhaps more generally useful are radio

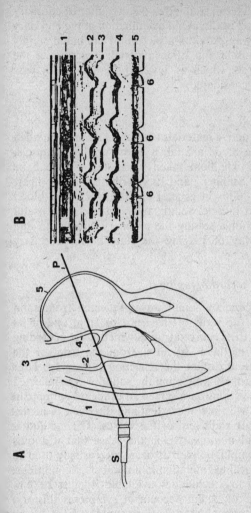

Fig. 13 Echocardiography.

A. Section through chest showing path of ultrasound wave.

B. Recording of echoes – showing movements of aortic wall and aortic valve during each heart beat.

Key: S = Source of sound.   2 = Near wall of aorta.   5 = Left atrial wall.
P = Path of sound.   3 = Aortic valve.   6 = Electrocardiogram marking heart beats.
1 = Chest wall.   4 = Further wall of aorta.

opaque dyes which can be injected directly into the coronary arteries. As stated in Chapter 4 examination of the coronary arteries in this way provides a picture of the blood supply to the heart muscle and often a detailed picture of the individual arteries which is invaluable when a by-pass grafting is being considered.

Scintigraphy

Certain radio active materials such as Thallium 201 when injected into the blood are taken up by the heart muscle. The amount of Thallium taken up in this way can be recorded by a "Scanner" and its distribution in the heart can be mapped. This in general corresponds to the blood flow in the heart muscle. Scintigraphy is therefore a useful indirect method of assessing the coronary circulation and an additional way of judging the state of the coronary arteries.

Ultra Sound. Echocardiography

Very high frequency sound waves reflected from solid objects such as the walls of the heart or from one of its valves return to their source at times which differ according to the distance of these structures from the front of the chest, i.e. the more distant the reflecting surface the later the time of return. By projecting the sound waves reflected from different positions on a screen an echocardiogram can be made which will show the extent and direction of movement of the heart walls and of the valves. The method is entirely safe and non-invasive in the sense that it avoids any internal manipulations. It is being increasingly used to supplement clinical examination in a number of conditions.

Despite so many techniques available it must be emphasised that a competent account of symptoms (history) and a careful physical examination, supplemented by an electrocardiogram and a plain X-Ray of the heart, remain the keystones of diagnosis of heart disease. They are fully adequate in the majority of cases. Physical examination requires special skills and should be undertaken by a trained person. Laymen should not attempt it. They can easily go wrong and can cause unnecessary worry. People who think they have heart disease must see a doctor.

7
THE CARE OF
YOUR HEART

PREVENTION OF HEART DISEASE

Prevention is always better than cure. This is particularly true of heart and blood vessel disease which in spite of the better treatment now available still cause by far the greatest number of deaths in the population. To say that prevention could ever be complete would be like offering a prescription for immortality. Much however has already been done to lessen the incidence of heart disease in young people and more could be done to offer better prospects of health to the middle aged and elderly. Rheumatic Fever for instance used to account for about one third of all cases of heart disease. Now thanks to better living conditions it is becoming almost a rarity in developed countries. The same is true of diphtheria because children can be immunised against it. German Measles during pregnancy is a major cause of congenital malformation but vaccination of susceptible mothers and of potential mothers to be is now possible and promises to reduce the disease if not to eliminate it.

High blood pressure and coronary heart disease remain and must be the next targets to attack. Both are partly familial or genetic in origin but both must owe something to the way of life in relatively wealthy societies. Until a better understanding of the factors involved indicates more radical solutions the main effort must be directed towards treating associated diseases such as diabetes, thyroid deficiency and kidney disease, and towards preventing an unhealthy way of life. Habits such as overeating, heavy cigarette smoking and a sedentary way of life, which are most closely associated, so often reflect personality reactions to the world about us and to a life style of chronic overstrain that it is difficult to consider them separately. In a perfect world their elimination would come about through changes in the outlook of society as a whole. These are unlikely in the foreseeable future and in practice it is up to the individual himself to decide to live healthily or to accept the possible consequences. He should decide early in life and should stick to his decision.

A HEALTHY WAY OF LIFE

This is not really a question of do's and dont's. Everyone must decide what suits him best. Perhaps it is easiest to recognise the warning signs which come when you are not living healthily. Are you losing your enjoyment of life at work or at play? A healthy person should look forward to both. Do you come home too tired and too preoccupied to enjoy your evening? Do you find it difficult to go to sleep and do you wake in the small hours and eventually oversleep in the morning? Are you drinking more, especially in the middle of the day, and are you smoking more cigarettes? What do you do at the weekend? Do you take regular exercise or follow some other form of recreation or do you just sit with a drink and a cigarette? Are you putting on weight? Are you losing your interest in sex? All these things can happen for a short time to anyone. Easing up will probably put them right. If they last more than a week or two you probably need a holiday. If they last much more than a month you ought to see your doctor. You may feel depressed but you may need to re-think your way of life. Is your work, business or your profession becoming too much for you; are you becoming cross and irritable with your colleagues and your family and difficult to work and live with? Do you forget things you ought to remember and are you finding it more difficult to take decisions? Are your colleagues or your family beginning to worry about you? Perhaps you are aiming too high. Perhaps you should delegate more and decide to accept the inevitable ups and downs of life, philosophically. Learn to relax, preferably with some demanding and enjoyable hobby.

Eating and drinking

So much conflicting advice has been given by experts that it is difficult to lay down hard and fast rules. Some have preached reduction of fats and cholesterol with almost obsessional determination, others have insisted on substituting unsaturated or essential fats for saturated fats, and still others have advised reducing the intake of sugar and other forms of refined carbohydrate. People with diabetes need appropriate dietary advice. Those with high levels of cholesterol (260 mgm per 100 cl.) from whatever cause need diets specially designed to lower them. These diets are otherwise unnecessary and the most important rule is not to overeat. The psychological effect of a good meal is not in doubt but the continued pursuit of "good eating" leads to trouble. So the first essential is to watch your weight.

A healthy person usually reaches his mature body weight in his middle twenties and maintains it fairly closely until old age when he begins to loose a little. Standard height/ weight tables give a fair guide to the average. Middle age spread is a social convention brought on by overeating and lack of exercise and not a biological necessity. Too often the process begins quite early when the pressures of business and professional life limit the time for regular exercise and when a loving wife takes over the kitchen.

What really matters is the total number of calories consumed and absorbed. Whatever their part in causing coronary disease may be, refined carbohydrates such as sugar are easily absorbed and offer the most certain way of putting on weight. It is not too difficult to avoid eating them in excess. Tea and coffee both taste better without sugar and fruit and puddings seldom need further sweetening. Sweets, soft drinks, sugar buns and sweet cakes should be taken sparingly. Those who are already accustomed to a sweet tooth can use a sugar substitute to bridge the gap. They may even find it so nauseating that they prefer to give up sweetening altogether. The direct rôle of dietary fats and especially of dairy produce is open to question. Rich fatty food undoubtedly encourages obesity and is better avoided. Fat meat, butter and cream are the foods to watch. Corn oil, sunflower and safflower oil, and soft margarines supply unsaturated and essential fatty acids and are better for cooking than saturated fats such as butter and lard. Meat should be lean and fish or chicken should be taken as regular alternatives. Roughage and dietary fibre helps to limit the absorption of carbohydrate and fat and is thought by some to protect against coronary artery disease. Its most certain rôle is in the prevention of intestinal disease. Taken as wholemeal bread, vegetable fibre, fresh fruit and bran-containing breakfast cereals it should have a regular place in a normal diet.

Alcohol is harmful in excess. Taken before meals it stimulates appetite and may aid the absorption of fats. It is in any case better avoided during working hours and kept for the evening. Moderate drinking such as a glass or two of wine with an evening meal is almost certainly harmless. It may even do good if it really does increase the proportion of high density lipoproteins in the blood as may be possible. Lunch time drinking of beer in pints is a social habit in men but it seldom stops at a pint when everyone has stood his round. If you must lunch with a regular drinking group drink in halves instead of in pints.

Cigarette smoking

Only too often this begins in teenagers who mistakenly think it is a sign of being grown up. The occasional cigarette becomes five, five a day become ten and ten become twenty before the victim realises that he is hooked. The habit gets worse when people are bored or under strain. The only safe course is not to start. Parents, schools and other educational bodies have a major responsibility, the exercise of which is of more likely use than high taxation and Government health warnings. If you have started keep to a maximum of five a day and watch carefully when you are bored or under stress. Fifteen a day or over is risky. If you cannot keep to five you should give smoking up altogether. Most people can do this if they try hard enough. Some give up at once; others keep careful count and reduce gradually. Often a minor illness makes cigarettes unpalatable. Cash in on it and give them up altogether. For those who need help special "stop smoking" clinics are available. A full and enjoyable life is probably the best antidote but if you have given up be careful not to start again when things go wrong. Some people on giving up smoking eat sweets as a substitute. This makes them put on weight but this can be corrected when the smoking habit is broken.

Exercise

There is much evidence to suggest that those who take regular vigorous exercise are relatively protected against coronary disease and particularly against fatal coronary attacks but there is still doubt whether exercise is in itself the crucial factor. Most people find the pattern of physical activity which suits them by the time they leave school. Those who do not want to take part in vigorous exercise or strenuous sport can keep perfectly healthy by the ordinary day to day physical activities of work and moving about as long as they do not put on weight by over-indulgence in food and drink. Provided that office life and car travel do not interfere with their normal habits there is no reason to convert them into reluctant athletes floundering perhaps incompetently, in a gymnasium or in a squash court or miserably jogging their measured urban miles.

It is always easier to keep fit than to get fit. Those who are accustomed to regular sport and exercise should try not to change their way of life. As one grows older competitive sport such as athletics and football become incompatible with a busy life but less strenuous activity can continue almost indefinitely provided people are healthy. Long distance running, rowing and sculling, squash racquets, tennis and cricket and so forth can all be undertaken with discretion but with enjoyment very nearly without limit. Whatever their intrinsic protective value they provide a sense of well being and a stimulating and absorbing mental and physical diversion usually in agreeable company. Those who do give up completely should beware of transferring their natural aggression to business or professional life, travelling always by car, allowing little time for relaxation and finding recreation in food, drink and tobacco. This is a path which leads quickly to a process of malignant ageing which is hard to reverse.

Those who have already travelled in this direction must however reverse, although carefully. Weight loss should be gradual, perhaps a stone in two or three months achieved by all round dietary restriction. Crash courses of orange juice and water and semi-starvation are not entirely free from risk, and there is reason to believe that too rapid weight loss can precipitate a coronary, possibly by excessively rapid mobilisation of stored fats. Exercise, at least within practicable limits, plays only a small part in weight reduction and should be resumed cautiously by those who have become unfit. Simple walking, climbing stairs or graded activity in a gymnasium to condition the body generally should precede any return to competitive sport. As you begin to do more your heart will certainly go faster (perhaps 150 beats a minute) and you will probably become breathless during exercise. At first this will go on for some time after the exercise but usually no longer than five minutes unless the exercise has been really strenuous – a three mile run perhaps. As you get fitter it will stop more quickly. If it does not you should see a doctor to make sure that nothing is wrong. If you get pain in the chest like Angina or you feel faint and likely to pass out you should see a doctor before taking any more exercise.

THE CARE OF A DAMAGED HEART

People with heart disease should always have expert medical advice. Two questions have to be answered. Is treatment necessary? What are the prospects for radical cure?

TREATMENT

Treatment is immediately necessary if the heart is failing or if it seems likely to fail. Sometimes if a major disorder of the heart beat is present this will require treatment straight away. Angina Pectoris, Coronary Thrombosis (Chapter 4), High Blood Pressure (Chapter 5) and Bacterial Endocarditis likewise need immediate medical attention.

Treatment for heart failure or threatened heart failure will vary according to the circumstances under which it has arisen. The objectives are always the same: to reduce the load on the heart, to treat any disorder or disease which may have brought on the failure, and to encourage the heart to perform better.

Any severe infection, particularly of the lungs, and also severe anaemia and thyroid disease, can cause a degree of heart failure but this will generally recover once the causal disease has been successfully treated.

Reducing the load on the heart

There are several ways of doing this. The first is Rest. A period of rest is nearly always advisable and in some cases necessary. For established heart failure rest at least initially means rest in bed, if necessary propped up on pillows or a bed rest to relieve breathlessness. Special beds have been designed to make this comfortable without causing obstruction to the blood flow from the lower limbs. This is necessary to avoid venous thrombosis and the consequent risk of pulmonary embolism. People being treated at home sometimes prefer to rest propped up in a comfortable armchair in their sitting room, if it can be conveniently arranged. Except immediately after a Coronary short walks to the lavatory are usually possible unless breathlessness is severe, but a bedside commode will be helpful.

Diet: There are no special instructions about food, but excess of heavy fluids such as soups and heavy vegetables often cause indigestion and are better avoided. Egg dishes, such as omelettes, fish, and chicken are usually preferable to meat. Cooking salt should be kept to the minimum needed to make food palatable and none should be added afterwards. Salt substitutes based on potassium rather than sodium are available if they are wanted. A glass of wine or moderate alcohol in some form is permissible.

Drugs: A number of different drugs are used. They act in different ways. Those which promote the excretion of salt (sodium) and water by the kidneys are known as diuretics and they are intended to reduce the circulating blood volume and so relieve the load on the heart. This is the quickest way of relieving congestion in the lungs and other organs such as the liver. Diuretics are usually taken once or twice daily by mouth as tablets. When very quick action is wanted as in cardiac asthma they can be injected into a vein. Diuretics often promote the excretion of potassium as well as sodium and this can become dangerous. To guard against it tablets of potassium (slow K) are generally taken at the same time.

Drugs of another kind reduce the load on the heart by dilating the smaller blood vessels. Dilatation of veins enables them to accommodate more blood and so lessens the amount of blood returning to the heart. Dilatation of the smaller arteries lowers the resistance in the circulation and lessens the force needed by the heart to maintain it.

Encouraging the heart to perform better

The most important stimulants to a failing heart are digitalis and drugs derived from it. Digitalis is an extract of the dried foxglove leaf which has been in use for nearly two hundred years. Its properties were first established by

William Withering, a Birmingham physician who recognised foxglove as the essential ingredient of a locally popular herbal brew used in Shropshire to cure dropsy. Ever since digitalis has been one of the mainstays of treatment for heart failure and for certain disorders of the heart beat such as atrial fibrillation and atrial flutter. Chemically synthesised components and other newer remedies have largely replaced the original preparation of foxglove leaf but in spite of certain drawbacks digitalis in some form still has an important place in the treatment of heart failure, particularly when it is caused by atrial fibrillation or mitral stenosis. Digitalis preparations are generally taken once or twice a day by mouth as tablets. They can be injected if very quick action is necessary. The chief disadvantage of digitalis is the narrow margin between a dose which is effective and a dose which can be harmful. Apart from digestive disturbances, such as nausea, loss of appetite and sometimes vomiting, digitalis can cause disorders of the heart beat which aggravate the heart failure which it is designed to treat. Dosage needs special care in children and the elderly and in people with very longstanding heart disease.

Disorders of the heart beat

Sometimes heart failure is brought on in people whose heart disease was previously giving them no trouble by *disorders of the heart beat*. Treating the disordered beat on lines to be described below will often restore the efficiency of the heart without the need for any further treatment.

Occasional disorders of the heart beat such as ectopic beats are unlikely to cause trouble and seldom need treatment. Paroxysmal disorders are likely to stop spontaneously and do not usually need treatment unless they are beginning to reduce the heart's efficiency. Those who have experienced many attacks sometimes have their own way of stopping them.

Atrial fibrillation and atrial flutter are generally associated with some form of heart muscle damage and are likely to cause some heart failure if they continue for any length of time. Both usually respond to drug treatment either with quinidine, a drug chemically related to quinine, or with a preparation of digitalis. This often takes time and it is generally quicker to treat them electrically under anaesthesia, a procedure which is in itself safe and often successful. Atrial fibrillation however is associated with a liability to form clots in the heart and a rapid return to normal beating can dislodge them and can cause embolism. The risk is greatest when mitral stenosis is present and when there has been longstanding fibrillation. Precautions can be taken to minimise the risk but the decision to convert to normal should be made only on experienced medical advice. If fibrillation resists conversion or if conversion is thought to be inadvisable the heart rate can be controlled by the use of digitalis with almost equally good results.

Ventricular tachycardias are so often associated with heart muscle disease that they nearly always need prompt treatment either by drugs or electrically.

Ventricular fibrillation must always be treated electrically at once. This is only possible in hospital or in a specially equipped ambulance.

EMERGENCY TREATMENT

Shock

Shock as explained in Chapter 3 is a severe and sudden failure of the output of the heart which occurs in conditions of acute muscle damage such as that caused by coronary thrombosis. It is a serious emergency which can be treated properly only in hospital. Many cases do occur there and most hospitals have special arrangements for dealing with it. Quite often however it occurs either at home or in the street. When it does an ambulance should be summoned immediately but in the meantime the layman should know what to do.

Prevention

If someone suddenly begins to feel ill and to complain of a pain in the centre of the chest like severe indigestion he is quite likely to be starting a coronary. This is the usual picture. The first thing to do is to try to prevent shock. Lay the patient flat, preferably on a hard surface, with his head only just off the ground (e.g. on a soft cushion) and keep him warm with a coat or a rug. Send for an ambulance.

Resuscitation and kiss of life

If in these circumstances the patient loses consciousness, goes a palish blue colour and stops breathing the heart has probably stopped. Strike a sharp blow across the centre of the chest, rather as if you were slamming a car door and then raise the legs to a right angle from the ground and keep them there for half a minute. This may start the heart again but if the patient does not begin to breath *you must start artificial respiration immediately.*

Kneel by the side of the patient. Tilt his head gently backwards and hold his jaw forward to clear the air way. Take a deep breath in and then breathe out firmly into the patient's mouth whilst *at the same time compressing his nose* with your thumb and forefinger (the kiss of life). This should expand the chest. Let it relax again and then repeat. Do this four times and see whether the patient recovers.

If not, start cardiac massage straight away. The patient must be on a hard surface. Kneel at his side and place both hands palm downwards one on top of the other on the lower part of the breast bone. Then, using the full weight of your body, compress the chest vigorously downwards (you can usually get nearly an inch of movement) once a second. After fifteen compressions stop and begin artificial respiration again for four more breaths. If there is no recovery waste no time but repeat the cardiac massage and then the artificial respiration again and keep on at it.

Resuscitation is hard work and two people are better than one. You must not give up even if the ambulance takes a little time to come. You never can tell when the heart will recover. Leave that to the doctors. When the patient recovers saliva and gastric contents are likely to be brought up. Turn his head to the side so that they can come out of his mouth and not go down into his lungs.

Is it a coronary or a faint?

Sometimes a coronary begins with shock and the patient faints immediately. An ordinary faint will probably come on slowly and the patient will feel it coming. As soon as he falls to the ground he will begin to recover. Also you may be able to feel his pulse which will be slow. If he *does not* begin to recover at once, assume it must be a coronary and proceed as above. However, do not forget that severe bleeding is another cause of fainting. Look for signs of this or of any accident which may have caused it. Try to control bleeding and get him to hospital at once.

Shock is the only heart emergency in which a layman's treatment, because it is immediate, may make the vital difference between life and death. Sometimes conditions such as the breathlessness of left heart failure can be temporarily helped by propping the patient upright with pillows and support for the back but the rule is that severe heart disease needs medical treatment as soon as possible.

Bacterial Endocarditis

A very important condition needing immediate treatment is Bacterial Endocarditis. The acute form occurs as part of a severe general illness and the treatment is by the antibiotics appropriate to the causal illness. Subacute Bacterial Endocarditis often occurs after dental extraction or after operations on the jaw and mouth. People with heart murmurs can usually be protected against the disease by giving antibiotics beforehand. Once the disease has begun treatment is needed urgently and should be given in hospital at least initially. It must be continued until all signs of active disease have disappeared. The difficulty is to recognise the condition in the early stages. People with valve disease or even with heart murmurs should see a doctor if they become feverish or generally unwell without any obvious cause for longer than a week. Treatment should be started even while steps are being taken to decide whether or not the disease is present.

Artificial pacemakers

An implanted pacemaker controls the heart's rate and is the accepted treatment for Stokes Adams attacks (p. 65). Pacemakers generally last for 6–12 years, with a clinical check at most twice a year. Inserted under the skin, usually near the right armpit, an electrode is fed from them through a convenient vein under x-ray control into the heart, so that the tip usually lies near the wall of the right ventricle.

Early pacemakers stimulated at a fixed rate. Sophisticated electronics now enable their stimulus to be inhibited by the electrical activity of the heart. This means after implantation they can be programmed to produce various stimulation rates depending on the heart's needs. Modern pacemakers are not upset by ordinary electrical apparatus unless it is faulty. Exposure to radar, microwave ovens or similar equipment needs caution.

RADICAL CURE OF HEART DISEASE: SURGERY

The outlook for congenital malformations and for valvular disease has been revolutionised by heart surgery. The first success was achieved when a ductus arteriosus (see Chapter 2) which had failed to close at birth was tied and obliterated and the circulation became normal. Later, fairly simple operations were introduced to relieve the obstruction and to mobilise the damaged valves in mitral stenosis.

The ability to stop the heart temporarily and to maintain the circulation artificially has since extended the scope and improved the quality of operations. Closure of abnormal communications within the heart has become increasingly effective and striking results have been achieved in complicated disorders such as those responsible for "blue babies".

Mitral incompetence and aortic valve disease still present problems but implantations of artificial valves and the successful grafting of human and pig's valves have gone some way towards solving them. By-pass grafts have already improved the quality of life and in some cases the prospects for survival of sufferers from Angina and promise to add a new dimension to treatment of coronary heart disease. Various mechanical devices to boost a failing heart have been tried but the most dramatic achievement has been the successful transplantations of whole human hearts.

Both the choice and the timing of surgical procedures require expert judgment. In congenital heart disease particular consideration must be given to the age and development of the child. Operation in infancy is not without risks but these are diminishing sharply and early operation to prevent irreversible structural damage is being increasingly undertaken. The time may even come when congenital heart disease may be accurately diagnosed before birth. A failing heart must generally be treated before surgery but this need not absolutely bar operation.

Heart transplantation being now technically feasible with successful transplants lasting for five year periods or more recorded, ethical considerations are paramount. Suitable "donor hearts" usually come from healthy young adults who have suffered brain damage, often as the result of injury. The supply is necessarily limited and precise and stringent conditions for a donor death must be satisfied in every case. Transplant operations are a great surgical achievement and demand specialised skills and experience but they are in some ways the least of the problems. Prevention of infection and avoidance of rejection of the alien heart continue to tax medical resources. Above all, the selected patients need determination and fortitude to enable them to undergo a difficult illness followed by continuing and sometimes prolonged drug treatment. With so many limiting conditions transplantation is likely to be reserved for fairly young people whose prospects for survival are small but who are likely to benefit from a new heart. In the face of bleak prospects the thought of a five year "reprieve", and perhaps considerably longer, may be welcome indeed. With the speed of medical advances now, worry over any longer period of time is likely to be removed by events.

LONG TERM MANAGEMENT

Once treatment for heart disease has become necessary it is likely to have to continue for some time, possibly permanently unless the underlying disease can be cured radically. Drugs must be taken regularly and their dose must be periodically regulated by a doctor. In addition some adjustment of the patient's way of life is almost certain to be necessary. Previously active people may find this irksome and frustrating. They must therefore learn to control their own activities and not be dependent on a number of do's and don'ts prescribed by their doctors.

To get the most out of life without overtaxing their heart, they must learn to recognise important symptoms and to know what they mean. Those being treated for heart failure should learn how much they can do without becoming uncomfortably short of breath. If they do become breathless they should stop what they are doing until the breathlessness wears off. If they become breathless when lying down or are woken up by breathlessness they may need stronger treatment and should tell their doctor about it. People with coronary heart disease should learn to recognise angina. If it comes on when they are doing anything they must stop until it goes off. Angina generally stops within five or at most fifteen minutes. If it lasts for more than half an hour it may be the start of a coronary. A doctor should be told at once or if that is impossible an ambulance should be sent for.

A fast heart beat during exercise is to be expected even in healthy people. In people with heart disease it may become uncomfortably fast (150 beats a minute). They should rest until it slows down again. If the beat is irregular when it has been previously regular a doctor should be told because there may be a disorder of rhythm needing special treatment. People recovering from a coronary can be helped by a period of graded exercise under supervision either in a hospital or a rehabilitation centre. This will not only enable them to learn what they can do safely but will often improve their performance considerably. There are no special rules about food and drink apart from not over-eating but those being treated for heart failure should avoid excessively salty foods. Generally there is plenty of salt in the cooking and it is a good rule not to add any more. Salt substitutes containing potassium instead of sodium are commercially available and may help some people.

Relatives and friends have an important part to play. They too must learn the guide lines. Their attitudes can make all the difference especially after a coronary when an over solicitous family can hinder a full recovery. Patients sometimes say that they would like to do more if only their wife wasn't watching them all the time as if their heart was a time bomb waiting for a convenient moment to blow up. Too much care is quite as bad as too little.

Children with heart disease sometimes present particular problems. Valvular disease and lesser congenital abnor-malities often cause no trouble and do not interfere with normal schooling and playing children's games. Special schools are seldom necessary except for those who are seriously handicapped. Competitive sport may be a problem for adolescents who should always have expert advice.

Improved surgical prospects have reduced the number of severely restricted children. Every effort should be made to allow them as normal a life as possible.

Fear of heart disease

A number of symptoms typically mistakenly believed to mean heart disease were mentioned in Chapter 3. Some of them were occasionally aggravated or even generated in the past by indecision on the part of doctors. Nowadays this should not happen and those who worry unnecessarily about their heart can usually be confidently reassured. They should always consult a doctor who can usually get to the bottom of their trouble.

Popular ideas about heart disease have undergone great changes recently and are still continuing to change. This book has attempted to describe the basis of heart disease and how it affects the ability of the heart to maintain the circulation. Though not necessarily serious in the life threatening sense, heart disease needs to be taken seriously. Diagnosis and treatment remain matters for doctors but explanations help patients to co-operate. By understanding they may come to terms with their disease and still get the best, or very nearly the best, out of life.

Doctors often use imprecise terms when talking to patients because they know how little most patients know about the heart and its working. Terms such as a "heart attack" can confuse unnecessarily while others like a "failing heart" frighten without meaning to. This book attempts by explaining them to put some of these things into perspective and perhaps thereby to relieve unnecessary fear.

EXPLANATIONS OF MEDICAL TERMS

Medical terms are often of either Greek or Latin origin. The reasons are largely historical but the terms are generally useful and have therefore been retained. Some traditional terms are imprecise in the light of modern knowledge and they have therefore been replaced in scientific use. However traditional usage still continues alongside and may cause confusion. These explanations attempt to clear up some muddling terminology as well as to simplify the meaning of those terms which are generally approved.

ALLERGY (literally altered reaction) usually means a widespread inflammatory reaction when the body is exposed to some substance to which it is sensitive either because of an inherited sensitivity or because sensitivity has been acquired after previous exposure. Ingested proteins, and bacterial infections are common causes. Rheumatic Fever is a characteristic example since infection of the throat of a sensitive person by a particular streptococcus provokes inflammation of joints and of the heart and pericardium without directly invading these structures.

AMINO-ACIDS are organic acids containing an amino-grouping which is a combination of Nitrogen and Hydrogen. There are many amino-acids in the body. Some are derived from food and others are directly synthesised by the body. They are essential components of protein and are a fundamental requirement of living tissue.

ANGINA PECTORIS (Greek: ankoné, a strangling sensation) is the constricting sensation, sometimes described as pain, in the chest when the blood supply and therefore the oxygen supply to the heart muscle is inadequate for the work that it is doing. Although generally the result of disease of the coronary arteries it can sometimes be the result of a poor coronary flow through healthy arteries.

ANTICOAGULANTS are drugs which interfere with the chemical components of blood clotting. Their chief value is in preventing thrombosis in veins. They are often used for this purpose before operations when thrombosis is a possible complication. They are also used in the early stages of a coronary attack but are usually discontinued when normal activity is resumed. Some drugs like aspirin interfere with platelet function – antiplatelet drugs. They are sometimes used in people who have recovered from a coronary in the hope of preventing further attacks.

AORTA (Greek: a strap) is the main systemic artery and takes oxygenated blood from the left side of the heart to all parts of the body. It is a long, arched strap-like vessel running upwards near the front of the chest as it leaves the left ventricle and turning backwards to descend close to the spine through the back of the chest and abdomen where it divides into two main branches to supply each of the lower limbs. (See Fig. 1.) Branches arise from the aorta at all levels to supply the different parts of the body. Two important branches (the carotid arteries) arise from the arched part of the aorta in the chest to supply the two sides of the brain. The terminal divisions of the aorta run downwards through the groin to the thighs, the back of the knees and the ankles (femoral arteries and branches).

ARRYTHMIAS (Greek: without rhythm) are disturbances of the rhythm of the heart beat either because of special circumstances influencing the normal pacemaker (sinus arrhythmia) or because the normal pacemaker control has been interrupted by a stimulus arising in another part of the heart. Sinus arrhythmia, found chiefly in young people, is caused by fluctuations of the heart rate in relation to breathing. Breathing in quickens the rate and breathing out slows it. The heart beat thus shows an alternation of faster and slower beats. The term dysrrhythmia (disordered rhythm) is sometimes used.

ARTERIOSCLEROSIS (Greek: hardening) is a general term used loosely to describe hardening of the arteries by ageing or by disease. (The term "arteriosclerotic" is sometimes used popularly to indicate senility.) Because of more precise definition of specific disease processes such as atheroma (see Chapter 4), and the arterial changes found with diabetes, high blood pressure, and other diseases, the term is scientifically obsolete.

ATHEROMA (see Arteriosclerosis).

ATRESIA (Greek: untraversed) refers to an unopened passage, e.g. an artery which has not admitted blood.

ATRIUM (Latin: hall or principle room in the house). The atria (plural) are the two receiving chambers of the heart. The right atrium receives blood from the great veins (the superior and inferior venae cavae) draining respectively the upper and lower parts of the body. The left atrium receives blood from the lungs via the pulmonary veins. The blood in the right atrium is therefore deoxygenated and the blood in the left atrium is oxygenated. The auricle (literally the ear) is a descriptive term properly applied to a small pouch on each atrium but it has sometimes been used to refer to the whole chamber. Atrium is proper current usage.

BACTERIUM (plural bacteria) is a general term for micro-organisms of different shapes and with different habits of growth and behaviour. Cocci (Greek: grain or berry) are round in shape. Staphylococci grow in clumps (Greek: clusters). Staphylococci usually cause disease such as boils or carbuncles, in the skin and the soft tissues. They also attack bones and cause abscess formation. They can affect other organs such as the lungs and the brain. Streptococci (Greek: twisted) grow in chains and are particularly responsible for disease in the throat, for Rheumatic Fever, and for certain forms of kidney disease.

BERI-BERI is caused by deficiency of thiamin, a member of the Vitamin B group. It is responsible for damage to nerves in the body as well as for damage to the heart muscle causing heart failure (see page 39). Mostly found in tropical countries because of inadequate vitamins in food. Excessive alcohol impairs the absorption of thiamin and is an important cause of deficiency in other parts of the world.

BRONCHITIS is an inflammation of the air passages (bronchi) in the lungs. Acute bronchitis produces an acute inflammation which usually recovers quickly. Chronic or long standing inflammation produces permanent structural changes which tend to narrow the air passages. Because of this air is trapped in the lungs which become over-distended (emphysema).

CALCIFIED Calcification means the deposition of chalk (calcium) in tissues usually occurring as a result of chronic inflammation (as in the pericardium) or of ageing or in the arteries affected by atheroma. It adds to the hardening process.

CALORIES are units of energy. One large kilo calorie is the amount of energy needed to raise the temperature of one kilogramme of water by one degree Centigrade. The calorie value of food varies with its nature. Approximately one gramme of protein produces 4.1 Calories. One gramme of fat produces 9.3 Calories and one gramme of carbohydrate produces 3.75 Calories. An average adult needs about 3000–4000 Calories daily for ordinary activity.

CARDIAC (Greek: the heart) is the adjective – pertaining to the heart.

CARDIOVASCULAR SYSTEM A general term to include the heart, arteries, capillaries and veins.

CHOLESTEROL circulates either in combination with a fatty acid or in free form. The total level of these two forms in the blood varies widely in healthy people. 150 mgs–250 mgs per decilitre are generally accepted as normal.

CORONARY The coronary arteries (Latin: a crown) encircle the heart like a crown. They are the first branches of the aorta and arise just beyond the flaps of the aortic valves. "Coronary heart disease" is disease of the heart muscle caused by disease of the coronary arteries. Sometimes called ischemic (Greek: deprived of blood) heart disease because the muscle is essentially deprived of blood. A "Coronary" or coronary attack is a popular term sometimes used by doctors to describe the clinical situation caused by acute damage to the heart muscle following obstruction usually by thrombosis of a coronary artery or one of its branches (Coronary Thrombosis).

COXSACKIE VIRUSES were first isolated in Coxsackie, a town in New York State, U.S.A. They usually cause an acute illness with fever and widespread inflammation of many parts of the body, particularly the muscles. The acute illness usually receeds fairly quickly but may leave permanent effects.

CYANOSIS (Greek: blueness) refers to the blueish colour affecting parts of the body in which the blood is poorly oxygenated. Two kinds of cyanosis are described. Central cyanosis affects all parts of the body and is the result of the circulation of inadequately oxygenated blood from the left heart through the systemic arteries. Peripheral cyanosis is caused by excessive local deoxygenation of the blood and usually affects the extremities of the circulation such as the lips, the ears and the nose, and the fingers. Central cyanosis is usually the result of congenital heart disease (see Chapter 2) or of chronic lung disease such as Bronchitis and Emphysema. Peripheral cyanosis is most often caused by stagnation of the circulation in cold conditions or by obstruction of veins, for example by a tight bandage on a limb.

DIASTOLE (Greek: tear open) is the period during which the heart muscle is relaxing with enlargement of the chamber concerned. In atrial diastole the atria receive blood from the systemic and pulmonary veins, in ventricular diastole the ventricles receive blood from the atria.

DILATATION means enlargement of a chamber or chambers of the heart usually because of increased pressure within them, together, in some cases, with weakness of the muscular walls. The capacity of the affected chamber and the overall size of the heart are increased and can be recognised fairly accurately by X-Rays. When a hypertrophied heart weakens the chamber affected dilates. Dilatation and hypertrophy therefore are often present together. See also under ENLARGEMENT.

Heart failure, except when it begins suddenly, is generally preceded by dilatation. A heart which is not enlarged is unlikely to fail.

DISEASE – DISORDER The term disease is used for when there is demonstrable damage in any part of the body. Disorder is used when a part of the body is working abnormally but is not necessarily damaged.

ECTOPIC (Greek: out of place) beats are caused by activation of the heart beat from a focus other than the normal pacemaker. They can arise in the atria, the atrio-ventricular node or the ventricles.

ELECTROCARDIOGRAM is a graphic record of the electrical changes occurring during the heart beat (see Chapter 6).

EMBOLISM (Greek: thrusting in) is the blockage or partial blockage of an artery by a portion of a recently formed thrombus which has been carried in the blood from another site. The usual site for the formation of the thrombus is either a deep systemic vein or the heart itself, either on a valve or in one of the atria. A characteristic example is embolism occurring in a pulmonary artery (pulmonary embolism). As a consequence of thrombus formation in a deep leg vein a portion of recently formed thrombus is detached and swept into the right atrium via the inferior vena cava (see Chapter 1). It then passes into the right ventricle which in turn expels it into the pulmon-ary artery. Once there it may obstruct the main artery or more often one of its branches.

EMPHYSEMA (Greek: blowing in) is a condition of the lungs in which air spaces are distended, generally as a result of longstanding narrowing of the air passages caused by chronic inflammation (chronic bronchitis). Emphysema may have serious effects on the pulmonary circulation. They include a raised pulmonary artery pressure (pulmonary hypertension) which often leads to right sided heart failure.

ENDOCARDITIS is inflammation of the endocardium or inner surface of the heart. The term in practice usually refers to one of the heart valves, e.g. Bacterial Endocarditis where a valve has become infected by bacteria.

ENDOGENOUS means something orginating from within the body. Endogenous metabolism is metabolism based upon substances generated within the body by its own chemical processes and not as directly supplied in food.

ENLARGEMENT of the heart is of two kinds, hypertrophy and dilatation. Hypertrophy (Greek: overgrowth) is a thickening of the muscular wall of one or more chambers of the heart, generally as a result of working permanently against increased pressure. This may be against high pressure in the arteries (high blood pressure) or against obstruction by damaged valves to the flow of blood through or out of the heart. Hypertrophied muscle can generally cope with the increased work but it demands a greater supply of blood than the coronary arteries can provide and eventually weakens. By itself hypertrophy increases the weight of the heart but hardly affects the capacity of the chambers concerned or the overall size of the heart. It usually produces an abnormal heart impulse which can be recognised by an experienced observer. It also alters the electrocardiogram.

ESTER Compound of organic acid and a hydrocarbon.

FAINTING ATTACKS cause loss of consciousness or a partial loss of consciousness because of temporary failure of the blood supply to the brain. Faints usually develop gradually over a minute or two, with a feeling of faintness or giddiness and general bodily weakness before the person falls or slides gradually to the ground. He becomes pale with a cold clammy sweat and a slow and often feeble pulse. As a rule improvement begins very soon after the person falls to the ground. Full recovery often takes time – feelings of faintness and coldness sometimes accompanied by vomiting may last for a quarter of an hour or longer. A number of heart conditions such as the onset of a coronary attack, a rapid disorder of the heart beat, or an obstructed aortic valve can cause temporary loss of consciousness but the majority of faints are not signs of heart disease. Overaction of the parasympathetic nervous system, associated with anxiety or tension is the commonest cause. Standing for long periods, particularly without moving the legs, is another common cause. It allows excessive amounts of blood to pool in the lower limb veins; this reduces the amount returning to the heart, and consequently the output from the heart. Faints of this kind are common in soldiers on parade. The development of a faint can often be prevented by lying flat on the ground or sitting in a chair with the head low between the legs.

HEART ATTACK is an imprecise and popular term without any medical meaning. It is sometimes used by doctors to describe to lay people any sudden disturbance of the heart's function ranging from the onset of a disorder of rhythm to a "coronary" or even a Stokes Adams attack (see page 65).

HEART BLOCK refers to delay or obstruction of the activating impulse as it passes from the pacemaker through the conducting system (for an account of the types and degrees of Heart Block see Chapter 3). Block does *not* mean that the flow of blood in the heart is blocked.

HYPERTENSION is a state of continued high blood pressure. Used by itself it refers to the systemic blood pressure. High pressure in the pulmonary circulation is referred to as pulmonary hypertension (see Chapter 5).

HYPERTROPHY see Enlargement.

INFARCTION (Latin: stuffing in) is a descriptive term based on the microscopic appearance of an area of tissue which has been suddenly and totally deprived of its blood supply. The area of tissue involved gradually dies off and becomes swollen because it is invaded by cellular elements of the blood from nearby healthy vessels. In due course scarring follows and the infarct shrinks. Infarction is nearly always caused by arterial obstruction, usually by thrombosis occurring directly in the artery concerned or by embolism. Thus a coronary thrombosis causes an infarct in the heart muscle. Doctors describe such events either in terms of the tissue damage, e.g. myocardial, cardiac or cerebral infarct, or in terms of what they believe to be the causal event, e.g. coronary thrombosis or cerebral embolism. Popular terms such as "a coronary" or a stroke refer to the resulting clinical disability.

JUGULAR (Latin: the neck or jaw) veins are the main veins in the neck. They carry blood from the head to join the superior venae cavae near its entry to the right atrium. In normal people sitting at an angle of 45° from the horizontal the deep veins in the neck are just visible and pulsate. The level of pulsation gives an indication of the pressure changes within the right atrium. A raised pressure in the jugular veins usually indicates that the right heart is failing.

THE MEDULLA is the lowest part of the brain and is the main centre for control of involuntary functions such as the heart rate, the blood pressure and breathing.

MYALGIA (Greek: muscle pain) implies muscle pain without reference to its cause.

MYCOPLASMA are micro organisms – midway in size between bacteria and viruses. They usually have no rigid walls. They are particularly liable to infect the lungs causing a characteristic inflammatory reaction known as mycoplasmal pneumonia.

MYOCARDIUM (Greek: heart muscle) Adjective myocardial.

PALPITATION is an imprecise term indicating unusual awareness of the heart beat. It may be caused by rapid, forceful, or irregular beating. Its significance depends entirely upon the cause. It is often experienced by healthy people during periods of stress or when frightened (palpitations). It is sometimes more obvious when lying down.

PATENCY is a state of being open. Used when a foetal communication in the heart remains open after birth when it should have closed, e.g. Patent ductus arteriosus.

PERICARDIUM, PERITONEUM, PLEURA These are thin membranous sacs investing or surrounding respectively the heart, the stomach and intestines and the lungs. Essentially each is a closed sac into which the organs in question have been thrust producing a situation similar to that produced by pushing the fingers of a glove inwards from the outside turning it half inside out. The cavity of the sac is in this way almost entirely taken up by the item being protected with the inner walls of the sac in apposition (touching each other). When these structures are attacked by inflammation inflammatory fluid is poured out between these walls thus separating them and causing a layer of fluid round the heart, the gut, or the lungs.

PERIPHERAL Applied to the circulation refers usually to small arteries, veins and capillaries in the systemic circulation.

PLATELETS Smallest cellular elements of the blood. Rhomboidal in shape. The site of much chemical activity they are of major importance in the control of haemorrhage and clot formation. Platelet clumping (aggregation) and platelet adhesiveness are essential to the process underlying thrombosis (see Chapter 4).

PROSTAGLANDINS A group of substances occurring in different parts of the body, the importance of which has been only recently recognised. Derived essentially from enzymatic oxygenation of a polyunsaturated fatty acid (arachidonic acid), they have major effects on platelet aggregation.

SPASM is generally applied to blood vessels and in particular to arteries which have narrowed as a result of contraction of their muscular wall with consequent reduction or even obliteration of their channel. Spasm probably occurs in arteries which are already damaged and is brought on by a number of different stimuli. It is usually temporary but may last long enough to cause damage to the tissue supplied by the artery.

STENOSIS (Greek: narrowing) is a term used when any structure such as a blood vessel, the channel between two heart chambers, or a portion of gut is narrowed and sometimes obstructed. E.g. mitral, aortic and pulmonary stenosis. Carotid (artery) stenosis.

STROKE is a popular term used to describe the effects of sudden damage to the brain caused by interference with its arterial blood supply, either by rupture or by blockage by thrombosis or embolism. The effects vary with the site and the severity of the damage. Commonly a part or parts of one side of the body, e.g. the face, arm or leg, are paralysed. A stroke usually causes sudden loss of consciousness.

SYMPATHETIC AND PARASYMPATHETIC NERVOUS SYSTEM sometimes together called the autonomic nervous system because it controls the action of parts of the body such as the heart and the gut which are not directly under voluntary control. The system is regulated by a centre in the medulla which is influenced partly by reflex action and partly by impulses from higher centres in the brain (central control).

Reflex action implies the control of nervous activity in response to incoming signals. A reflex arc consists of an incoming nerve which conveys signals into the brain or the spinal cord from the part of the body where it is situated. These are relayed centrally to a corresponding outgoing nerve which responds either by increasing or by decreasing the number of impulses going back to the target organ. The autonomic nervous system works by releasing chemical substances in the organs which it controls. These are taken up by special receptor cells. Sympathetic nerves (except in one or two areas such as some of the fibres in muscle, where they release acetylcholine), release adrenaline and nor-adrenaline. Parasympathetic nerves release acetylcholine. Sympathetic nerves are therefore sometimes spoken of as adrenergic except where they release acetylcholine, and parasympathetic nerves are sometimes called cholinergic. A degree of permanent control of the autonomic system is exercised largely by the lower centre in the brain. The action of adrenaline and acetylcholine on the heart and blood vessels is discussed in Chapter 1. The actions of these substances can be prevented by drugs known as nor-adrenergic antagonists. Propranolol, used in the treatment of high blood pressure and angina pectoris, works in this way.

SYSTEMIC CIRCULATION is the circulation to and from all parts of the body. The aorta and its branches and the superior and inferior venae cavae and their tributaries are respectively the outgoing and incoming vessels of the systemic circulation. The systemic circulation is sometimes known as the greater circulation to distinguish it from the lesser or pulmonary circulation which takes blood through the lungs for oxygenation. The lungs themselves receive their own blood supply from the systemic circulation.

SYSTOLE (Greek: contraction or collection) denotes the period when the heart muscle is contracting. Atrial systole is the contraction of the atria and ventricular systole the contraction of the ventricles. The heart beat which can be felt in the chest is caused by ventricular systole. During atrial systole blood is forced out of the atria into the ventricles. During ventricular systole blood is forced out of the ventricles into the aorta and pulmonary artery.

TACHYCARDIA (Greek: swift) means rapid heart beating. It may indicate any increase in heart rate, usually to over 100 beats per minute. The term is chiefly used to describe paroxysmal disorders of the heart beat. *Bradycardia* (Greek: slow), usually applied to rates below 60 per minute.

THERAPY (Greek: care, service) Process of care and treatment. Adjective – therapeutic.

THROMBOSIS is the process of thrombus formation. See Chapter 4.

TOXOPLASMUS Widespread disorder caused by parasites and having a number of different manifestations. People in many communities are affected without showing any sign of disease.

TRYPANOSOMES Protozoa carried by the tsetse fly and causing sleeping sickness in Africa.

UMBILICAL CORD is the main connection between the mother and the unborn child in the womb. It carries deoxygenated blood to the placenta (this is what becomes the after birth) in the umbilical arteries and receives oxygenated blood back into the foetal circulation from the umbilical veins. The cord has to be tied off at birth.

(HEART) VALVES are thin freely mobile flaps roughly triangular in shape. Each valve has either two or three flaps (cusps). They are attached at their base to the walls of the channels which they control, i.e. to the walls of the heart at the junction between the atria and the corresponding ventricles and to the walls of the aorta and pulmonary artery. The flaps project freely into the channel when open and come together to close it. (See Fig. 4.)

VIRUSES are the smallest form of microbial life and consist basically of nuclear material (ribo- and deoxyribo-nuclear acids). They pass through the smallest physical filter and are therefore sometimes know as filterable viruses. Responsible for a wide spectrum of disease of which the common cold, influenza and poliomyelitis are perhaps the most well known.

INDEX

OUR PUBLISHING POLICY

HOW WE CHOOSE

Our policy is to consider every deserving manuscript and we can give special editorial help where an author is an authority on his subject but an inexperienced writer. We are rigorously selective in the choice of books we publish. We set the highest standards of editorial quality and accuracy. This means that a *Paperfront* is easy to understand and delightful to read. Where illustrations are necessary to convey points of detail, these are drawn up by a subject specialist artist from our panel.

HOW WE KEEP PRICES LOW

We aim for the big seller. This enables us to order enormous print runs and achieve the lowest price for you. Unfortunately, this means that you will not find in the *Paperfront* list any titles on obscure subjects of minority interest only. These could not be printed in large enough quantities to be sold for the low price at which we offer this series. We sell almost all our *Paperfronts* at the same unit price. This saves a lot of fiddling about in our clerical departments and helps us to give you world-beating value. Under this system, the longer titles are offered at a price which we believe to be unmatched by any publisher in the world.

OUR DISTRIBUTION SYSTEM

Because of the competitive price, and the rapid turnover, *Paperfronts* are possibly the most profitable line a bookseller can handle. They are stocked by the best bookshops all over the world. It may be that your bookseller has run out of stock of a particular title. If so, he can order more from us at any time—we have a fine reputation for "same day" despatch, and we supply any order, however small (even a single copy), to any bookseller who has an account with us. We prefer you to buy from your bookseller, as this reminds him of the strong underlying public demand for *Paperfronts*. Members of the public who live in remote places, or who are housebound, or whose local bookseller is unco-operative, can order direct from us by post.

FREE

If you would like an up-to-date list of all paperfront titles currently available, send a stamped self-addressed envelope to
ELLIOT RIGHT WAY BOOKS, BRIGHTON RD.,
LOWER KINGSWOOD, SURREY, U.K.